Hanging On

Hila Colman

HANGING ON

New York ATHENEUM 1977

Library of Congress Cataloging in Publication Data

Colman, Hila.
    Hanging on.

    1. Cerebrovascular disease—Biography.
2. Colman, Hila. I. Title.
RC388.5.C64   362.1'9'8109   76-58382
ISBN 0-689-10788-9

Published simultaneously in Canada by McClelland and Stewart Ltd.
Manufactured by American Book-Stratford Press, Inc.
Saddle Brook, New Jersey
Designed by Harry Ford
First Edition

This is Limey's book
and our children's
and their children's

Hanging On

Part One

You paid attention to Limey. We all did. He made his presence felt. His very existence in a room, in a house, made all of us, his grandchildren, his sons and daughters-in-law, his friends, aware of his sensibilities. Women especially, the most fiercely independent of them, including me, his wife, wanted to please him. Hostesses urged him to take the most comfortable chair, they planned elaborate meals around his preferences, they worried that he not be bored, and when, inevitably, the most attractive women gravitated toward him, everyone was relieved. If Limey was having a good time, the party had to be a success.

On the surface it might seem unlikely that Limey's personality would endear him so wholeheartedly to so many people. He had a talent for delivering opinions as if from the Mount, and even with his encyclopedic mind, his facts were not always totally accurate. I think that Limey's lovable quality came at least in part from the fact that he was constantly astonished that anyone would listen to him. He honestly believed that what he said could not possibly affect another person's thinking or actions, nor was he at all aware of the authority with which he spoke. And on those rare occasions when he was proven wrong—a glorious victory for the person who had bothered to check his facts—Limey welcomed the new information with an eager, childish delight. This of course was a letdown for the victor, but you couldn't help being warmed by this man's lack of self-awareness and his earnest love for the accumulation of knowledge.

One day Limey came upon me diligently snipping off all the blossoms from the annuals we had laboriously transplanted together. "What are you doing that for?" Limey demanded. "I came out to admire them."

"You told me to. You once said the plants would be healthier."

Limey couldn't believe I had taken him at his word. Then he gave me his most disarming smile. "Maybe. But they'll be all right as they are. They look so colorful." But even he could not undo what he had once stated with such conviction, and I was compelled to snip until the last blossom was gone.

Limey's wide range of knowledge did not always make him an easy man to live with. While it was beautifully convenient to have so much information at hand—how to make a béchamel sauce, household lore, names of the plants in the woods, an exact quote from the Bible, where the Aru Islands were, who wrote the Rubaiyat, or who had been Secretary of State under Woodrow Wilson—the precision he expected in return was often more than I could deliver. My mind runs more to fiction than to fact. But our differences had their advantages: although they made for strenuous arguments, we were not competitive.

In spite of Limey's sophistication, he was a domestic man of simple tastes. He could enjoy a hamburger as well as a gourmet feast, but the meat had to be succulent, rare, and put on a toasted "fit-to-eat roll, not one of those damned, plastic buns."

Limey loved our home, and he delighted in every improvement, whether it was a new frying pan or a new terrace. He loved to sit by the fire with a drink at hand and read, or just to sit. He took pleasure in words, in walking in the woods to find the first morels, in shopping for food, in picking up shells on the beach, in conversation with friends. He carried baby pictures of our two sons in his wallet, although he insisted that you brought children up to leave home. But when they did grow up and leave he missed them sorely, and was as eager as I for their visits, swelling with pleasure when they greeted him with an affectionate hug and a kiss rather than a handshake.

This was Louis, my husband, nicknamed Limey. The name originated when, at about seventeen or eighteen, he signed up as a mess boy on a ship sailing to the east coast from California. Limey's story was that the crew did not know what to call him. According to him, they couldn't say, "Come here, Louey," as on shipboard, so he said, a

Louey was a lad who serviced the men sexually. So because of his odd accent—he spent his first six years in Switzerland speaking only French, and then learned English in Canada—they hit on the name Limey. The name stuck, I suspect, mainly because he never liked the name Louis. My husband: complicated, rigid and uncompromising in many areas, simple in his tastes, highly intelligent and filled with knowledge both useful and esoteric, not an easy person but lovable and tender, a private person, capable of extremes of temper and passion, and, on a cold, raw day in January 1975, driving me out of my mind.

The house was too small for his pacing. Back and forth, back and forth. I could feel the tension seeping through the walls into my study, where I was trying to work. God damn, why couldn't he relax?

If I had put the question to Limey he would have laughed as he had five years earlier at the doctors. "To ask someone to relax can only produce the opposite."

That had been on the occasion of his first "incident"— what the doctors called "a cerebral accident." I don't know why no one had said "stroke" to us. Perhaps because it had come upon him gradually over a period of several days, not suddenly, the way most people think of stroke. At that time he was a medical writer for a large pharmaceutical company in New York, and we kept a small apartment in the city, which Limey used during the week. One Friday night he came home to our house in Connecticut, where I stayed a good deal of the time, looking gray and very tired. "I had to pull over to the side of the road," Limey said. "On the highway I felt myself losing control of the car. But I managed to get home all right, as you see," he added.

Neither one of us was particularly alarmed, and we put it down to fatigue. Limey rested over the weekend and was up fresh and early Monday morning to go back to the city. "Be careful with the driving," I said.

Monday afternoon he called to tell me that he was going into the hospital for some tests. He had had trouble driving again, and had called our good friend Dr. Toby Wolf, a neurologist, who told him to have someone bring him to his office. Limey assured me that it was nothing serious, but I got down to New York in a hurry.

I went up to the hospital with Limey and we were both cheerful when I left him there. The next afternoon when I went back, Toby was there to greet me. "Well, he doesn't have a brain tumor," he said.

I stared at his smiling face in a state of shock. "Brain tumor?" I shrieked. "Is that what you were looking for?"

"We had to rule that out," he said blandly.

"Then what is it, for God's sake?"

"We don't know yet."

Limey was sitting up in bed looking cheery and fascinated, as he always was when acquiring new medical information. I can't say that he enjoyed having the brain scans and the EKG's and God knows what all they were putting him through, but he was exceedingly good-natured about them. Interested in an objective way, as a person who enjoys research would be.

But the next few days didn't turn out to be all that

cheery and fascinating. The tests and X rays showed that Limey had a blockage in his left carotid artery, one of the two main arteries in the neck that carry blood to the head. This plaque, as the doctors called it, affected his peripheral vision on both sides, his sense of space and balance, and, in particular, his right arm and leg. They didn't keep him in the hospital for long; the main medication, they said, was rest and time.

Back home in Connecticut, Limey had one frustrating experience after another. He found that he could not write or eat with his right hand. He had no control, and if he held a glass in it he would as likely drop it as not. He could not drive, and in the house everything had to remain strictly in its place, although even then he often thought he was bumping into something when he wasn't. But what really frustrated him the most was getting dressed. He had difficulty finding the sleeves to put his arms through, he put shirts on backward, he had trouble managing buttons, and he could not tie shoelaces. From then on Limey wore only laceless soft shoes he could slip his feet into easily. I did not offer to help him get dressed, although the process was nerve-wracking to watch, and I quickly absented myself from that scene. He himself knew that he had to work at it, and he did. Little by little Limey's coordination improved—although it was a slow, painful process that never became normal—and on the occasions when he had to wear a tie, he insisted on knotting it himself and he did a respectable job.

He had to quit going to work, which was a big financial blow, but we gave up the New York apartment, and managed. Eventually Limey learned to work on an electric typewriter, a machine he had previously shunned (an old newspaperman, he preferred an ancient portable). He tried to use his left hand as much as possible, but he also used his right hand more than he had in the beginning.

I did not cater to Limey's handicaps. We lived as we had before, fighting, loving, eating, drinking, reading, walking, entertaining, going out. The big difference was that Limey was home, not earning any money (he did get a small pension from his last job, and his social security, and I continued to write my books for children, as I had for many years), and he could not do all the things he had done before. But I did not think of him as an invalid in any way, and in fact he was not, although he tired easily and almost always rested during some part of the day. He also spent long hours at his typewriter writing only what he wanted to write, poetry and his memoirs. He wrote hundreds of pages about his childhood and youth, and after all those years, finally tried to resolve his feelings about his family, particularly his parents, both of whom had died many years before I knew him. He had rather a stockpile of ambivalent emotions to sort out: his fanatically religious Presbyterian preacher father had made him stay indoors an entire summer at the age of twelve to memorize the catechism. At the end of the summer, however, when his gentle, suffering mother was told to give him the test, she had allowed him to look over her shoulder at the text. He had four sisters, and an older brother, Morris, to whom he had turned when he had left home at sixteen—or, as Limey claimed, had been thrown out by his father for stubbornly refusing to admit to a lie of which his father had wrongly accused him.

I had a terrible time adjusting to Limey's being home all day. I am a restless writer, and alone in the house I had been in the habit of getting up from my typewriter frequently to roam around the house, often to do some mechanical job in the kitchen, not wanting to talk to anyone, my mind on my book. Limey liked to spread his *New York Times* out on the big kitchen table and to read it there, simultaneously keeping his sharp and often critical eye on what I was doing at the counter. But I protested. My culinary shortcuts were none of my perfectionist husband's business. So the kitchen was designated out of bounds for Limey.

Actually we worked out a good life for ourselves. Because of Limey's poor circulation he could not take the cold weather, and for four years we spent the winter months in Mexico. Mexico was not expensive, and by closing our house and avoiding the rising costs of fuel and utilities, we were able to afford it. However, in 1975 we decided to try Sarasota, Florida, for our winter sojourn.

Florida had been my idea and Limey had to be persuaded. He had been to Florida before I knew him, and hated it. "Flat and dull," he said. But I had a vision of white beaches, sparkling water, and freedom from coping with mountainous roads and a foreign language and a very long trip (I did not fly). But to persuade Limey to do something that he initially resisted was a hazardous venture.

A few weeks before we were to leave, Limey was annoyed because his typewriter was being repaired. He paced the floor, furious because he was not working on notes he wanted to take with him to Florida. Limey had never outgrown his puritanical upbringing of Work before Play, and by God, you've got to get that work done no matter what. Although only rarely did he say, "I don't have much time," I knew he was racing against time to put down everything he wanted to say. Yet his compulsive work, the long hours sitting at his desk, worried me. He wasn't getting enough exercise and he was smoking too much. But how does a wife straddle the line between not being a nag and trying to persuade a stubborn husband to take care of his health?

In retrospect I like to think that the sense of doom I had felt all that fall about our winter in Florida was a mystical gift I had acquired, but I fear it was nothing more than a familiar uneasiness about whether or not Limey was going to like it: was the apartment we'd picked from a bunch of folders sent to us by the Chamber of Commerce going to live up to its promise, was the weather going to be as comfortable as at Cuernavaca, was the ambiance going to be interesting, was Limey going to thrive, to enjoy the people and the surroundings, or was it all going to be a flop?

Wrongly or rightly I felt it was all on my head. It would never occur to Limey to hold me responsible, but dammit, it was that same hard-to-define quality of Limey's that made you want to make the act of living less of a burden for him. You—I—wanted to smooth away the rough edges, to lighten the intensity of his awareness and his reaction to his surroundings. Fond of saying, "I don't care, you decide," he really did care. He was not indifferent. He reacted to the comfort or discomfort of a chair, to how a bed was made, to the lighting in a room, to the feel of material. And Limey had a talent for putting his finger immediately on the flaw. He was offended by wrinkled sheets, by jarring voices, by jargon, the misuse of language, by anything shoddy or ersatz. He was not good at faking; his feelings showed. But what he did enjoy, he enjoyed thoroughly. As a good friend of ours said, "When you did something for Limey that pleased him, it really made you feel good, you felt an immense satisfaction."

If there is such a person as an ideal wife, I was not it. Far from it. The daughter of a successful businesswoman (who died way before women's lib was invented), I was brought up to believe that a woman had to be independent, to earn and have her own money and her own point of view, that housework was something one paid someone else to do, and that to spend one's life catering to a man's whims was quite ridiculous. But, unfortunately, as with a first baby or death, few of us are prepared for love. Loving Limey was not easy. My rational mind told me that Limey's sensitivity, the burden of pain that he carried through life, was not of my doing (he quite rightly laid a lot of the pain on his tyrannical father), yet I could not push aside my own driving need, because I did love him, to make life work for him—and when catastrophe hit us, this need became central to me. I was a woman struggling to maintain her own identity, her own independence, and at the same time wanting, needing, to make her man happy—a foolish word that Limey always said had no meaning, and perhaps he was right. Maybe, after all, happiness is only the absence of pain. The words "cater to" have the ring of humiliation, of performing a lowly service—yet to do something for a person one cares about seems so obvious and natural that I get annoyed and confused by those who weigh it down with talk of sexism and chauvinism.

Fine words. But I was not all that successful in straddling that slim line between feeling responsible for Limey (why should I? He was a big, grown man) and telling myself, hell, asking a man to spend a winter in Sarasota wasn't the worst thing in the world, and why shouldn't we do what I wanted for one year? Not surprisingly, there was tension in our house. Limey and I had always been capable of trapping ourselves into passionate arguments about absurd trivia such as who should call the plumber or what pot made the best coffee. But it seems to me that at that time we weren't arguing so much as warily keeping a watchful distance and nursing our own nerves.

Later, I asked Dr. Wolf whether studies had ever been made on the life patterns of patients directly before suffering a major stroke. Had they been under particular stress or tension? He said that some research had been done in that area, but that the data was not easy to come by. "But even if we knew," he told me, "the big question that remains is why one person under tension may get a stroke and the next one not." Limey had none of the publicized signals. He never had high blood pressure—it was always low, if anything; he had no history of heart ailment; he did not have a high level of cholesterol or triglycerides in his blood. He did have poor circulation in his feet—they were always cold—and he was a heavy smoker. Perhaps more than anything he lived hard. Limey was an intense man, and everything mattered to him. He was never one of those myopic men who paid no attention. He courted involvement, in the details of our household and in the activities of our family. After that first stroke, when his balance was shaky, he never avoided the rushing on-slaught of his five young grandchildren: their mother and I would watch with apprehension the noisy whirlwind head in his direction, and Limey would simply stand ab-solutely still, resting on his cane, a smile on his face, and make no concession to his infirmity. They never knocked him down.

One of the things I often thought about, but never got a medical opinion on, was how long it had taken that plaque in Limey's carotid artery to form. Had it been a gradual process over a few years, many years? Surely it didn't accumulate overnight. I still wonder about it, be-cause Limey was never good at visualizing space. When-ever we had to move furniture around, Limey had no concept of where anything would fit. We once had a rous-ing argument about a beautiful old six-foot table I wanted to buy for our kitchen.

"You're crazy," Limey told me. "It can't possibly get into our kitchen."

In his methodical way Limey measured out the kitchen floor before the table was allowed into the house. With six chairs around it, the table was not at all crowded. The question that bothered me was had Limey been hit in his weakest, most vulnerable spot, or was it vulnerable because the plaque in his blood had been forming? Or was it all irrelevant? Who knows?

The day finally came when our bags were packed, the rugs sprinkled with mothballs, our big black poodle taken to the kennel, and the plumber summoned to turn off the water. (*I* called him.) We were going to have dinner and spend the night with our neighbors and good friends, Bob and his wife, and leave early the next morning. The great thing was that Bob had decided to drive down to Florida with us. Bob is one of those rare humans who, when he is doing you a favor, convinces you he is doing something for himself. I will never know whether Bob truly wanted to spend a few days in Florida (his plan was to stay for the weekend and fly home) or whether he came because he could spell me with the driving and also make the trip smoother for Limey. But for whatever reason, his being along turned out to be one of the few lucky breaks we had.

We packed the car with suitcases (clothes for three or four months), typewriters, folios of work, a bag of books, bourbon and snacks for afternoon arrival at motels, raincoats, overnight bags, and a picnic basket with our favorite on-the-road lunch of cold chicken, fresh rolls, tomatoes, and a bottle of white wine. We did not travel light.

It was a clear, bright, cold day in January, and the minute we were off on Route 84, to take the Tappan Zee Bridge across to New Jersey, all tensions vanished. We were really going to a warm, sunny place, directly on a beach, and I had a letter in my pocket from friends in Sarasota saying that they had checked out our apartment and found it clean, comfortable, and well equipped.

I like journeys. I don't like being hurled swiftly through the air from one place to another. I like to savor the trip, to relax, to think about where I am going, and to see what I can along the way. Happily Bob chose to take the first shift, driving what I considered the most unpleasant part of the road, the New Jersey Turnpike. I was settled in front, next to him, with the maps on my lap, and Limey had the back to himself. Limey and I rarely talked much in a car, but we had a habit of reaching over to pat each other, and now I was able to reach back every so often and hold his hand for a minute or two. I felt good. It had all worked: I went over our luggage in my mind and I didn't think we had forgotten anything; our house had been left in good shape, telephone disconnected, forwarding of mail arranged for, bills paid, letters answered, our 1972 Plymouth tuned and fitted with new tires—we were on the road with a fine driver at the wheel. I could relax.

We picnicked on a dirt side road, and finally stopped for the night someplace in Virginia I think—or maybe it was Maryland, I don't remember. Limey was tired, but that did not seem extraordinary. I was tired too, as I believe anyone would be after three hundred miles or more of driving. We had a couple of drinks in our motel room before going downstairs to one of those dreary restaurants one finds in or near every motel on the way south. None of us felt like bothering to look around for something better.

I was rather relieved, for once, to hear Limey expounding in his usual extravagant, explosive way about bad food. "This plastic stuff is inedible," he declared, cutting into a piece of tough, stringy meat. "And do they call this salad?" he demanded scathingly of the iceberg lettuce the waitress put before him. "This food, if you can call it that, is an insult." His resonant voice boomed out, to Bob's discomfort, but I was glad that Limey's fatigue was not sufficient to impair his normal uninhibited style.

After dinner we went to our rooms, agreeing to get up no later than seven to make an early start. I rather like motel rooms. I like to open up all those drawers to see what, if anything, is inside, to look at where the marker on the Bible has been left, and to wonder who had been reading it. Someone at one time had bothered to design that room, to put together all that ugliness, to select the conglomeration of colors and the dreadful pictures on the walls. What was in his mind? Yet he had achieved a certain comfort, with lights over the beds and lots of mirrors and hangers that cannot be stolen but also do not fall down. Those ample twin double beds are one of the better ideas. Limey was able to stretch out on his (he loved large

beds) and go to sleep, while I could read without disturbing him.

Wednesday, another uneventful but pleasant day on the
road. The landscape was becoming more interesting, and
prettier; Limey was still fatigued but in good spirits. We
stopped at one of the places advertising cigarettes at bargain prices. It had looked okay from the outside, but inside it was like going into a spooky underground cave
that possibly doubled as a brothel. It was dark, with all
manner of objects hung from the ceiling: beads, shells,
junk jewelry, nuts, a good many of them covered with
cobwebs that brushed against our faces. There was not an
inch of space—tables, walls, a dirty glass counter—that
was not covered with something to sell. Behind the
counter sat an old witch with long, straggly gray hair
who looked at us with an expectant smile on her wrinkled face. "I have some beautiful rings," she said, point-
ing to a tray of what looked like dime-store items to me.

"No, thank you." I wanted to get out fast. But not
Limey. I could see his blue eyes melting, and I could read
his mind: this poor old woman sitting here alone all day
with all this junk, waiting for someone to stop . . . I
waited outside and was not surprised when Limey came
out, not only with cigarettes, but with shells and rocks
(the kind you could pick up anywhere) and some awful
postcards. He was sorry he hadn't had more money and
that she couldn't cash a twenty-dollar traveler's check.

We discussed going out of our way to see Charleston,
decided against it, and opted instead for looking at the
newly restored waterfront buildings in Savannah,

Georgia. I had read an article in the *New York Times* that made a stop there sound worthwhile. We arrived sometime Thursday morning, after another night at an undistinguished motel. Savannah's waterfront was something of a disappointment. Perhaps because it was morning, the shops didn't look open, and many buildings were still unfinished. At any rate, we didn't stay around for long, but continued on our way.

As we drove toward Florida—my first experience at it—I had to remind myself as we passed other cars and campers with northern license plates that we were not just another statistical couple, unhappily labeled Senior Citizens, in search of moderate living and sunshine. We were Limey and me (and younger Bob), professional writers, with no intention of ever becoming Senior Citizens regardless of our ages. I told myself that we were not going to Miami, that we were going to swim and walk and work, that we were going to theaters and operas, and that we were as alive and interested and engaged with each other and with life as we had always been.

My gloomy forebodings had vanished and did not even return on Thursday evening when Limey seemed a little unstable when he walked. He had gotten into the habit of using a cane, one specially designed to fit into his left hand, but even with that he was stumbling. "It's probably from sitting in the car too much," I said. "Your legs must be stiff." In view of the poor circulation in his legs, that seemed a plausible explanation. However, his face did look drawn and tired. With his gray hair receding on his long, narrow, well-shaped head, his varicolored but predominantly gray mustache and Vandyke beard, his very bright blue eyes gave the only spot of color to a somewhat colorless face. But I am not the one to describe Limey's looks. I think he had a beautiful face and body. He was particularly proud of his feet. His toes were straight, "not curled up because of lousy shoes," he boasted. He had extraordinarily fine skin that could take little sun, a tall, narrow-hipped, somewhat gaunt physique, and a mobile face that made no attempt to hide his feelings.

That evening he was very fatigued and seemed preoc-cupied. Bob was the one who was worried. "Would you rather turn back and go home?" he asked Limey. "We can, you know."

"No, of course not," Limey told him. "I'll be all right when we get there. It's just this damn trip."

"Just one more day," I said. "Next year you had better fly wherever we go." Next year, next year . . . a lifelong disastrous pattern of projecting into the future.

We weren't pushing hard to make time. Four days to get to Sarasota meant averaging around three hundred miles a day, which allowed for plenty of stops along the way, and quitting in the afternoon before it got dark. As a matter of fact, I had told the woman who owned the apartment we were renting that we would not arrive until sometime on Saturday. On Friday afternoon, however, we were less than a hundred miles from Sarasota, and we all felt we would much prefer spending the night in our own place. So we stopped and I called up Mrs. Vogel. She said the apartment was ready, she was just giving it a last-minute going-over. That sounded great to me. We had no

difficulty finding our number on Gulf of Mexico Drive on
Longboat Key, although it was quite dark when we
arrived.

We were not disappointed in what we found. A motel
of not more than five or six units, directly facing a lovely
beach, lounge chairs on a pretty garden and lawn outside
our door. The apartment itself had a screened porch, an
airy living room (with a couch that turned into a bed for
Bob), a dining area, bath, bedroom with twin beds and
cross ventilation, a good-sized and well-equipped kitchen
and a large pantry. We couldn't miss—we were going to
have a fine winter here.

Limey agreed to sit down while Bob and I unloaded the
car. We left our bags unopened, but it was well past nine-
thirty when we went in search of a place to eat. Most were
closed or closing, but on Siesta Key we found a rather big,
gloomy, nightclub-type restaurant where we were told we
could get food. We had a not very good but very expensive steak dinner (I had been longing for the fresh fish
which I had associated with Florida), and Bob and I consumed rather a large quantity of brandy. Limey, who
usually had a good appetite for food and liquor, was not
much interested in either.

When we got back to the apartment Limey had a little
difficulty getting undressed, he was fumbling and im-
mensely annoyed with himself, and that night I did help
get him into his pajamas and into bed. His frustrated
"goddammits" were familiar, and I was still seeing only a
temporary setback, a result of the weariness of the trip.
The five years since Limey's first episode had not been

straight, smooth sailing. There had been many ups and downs, good days and bad days, depending a great deal on how tired he was, or on the weather, or on his mood; his mental state greatly affected his physical abilities. I had seen him take long, rough walks, without a cane, through the woods one day, and appear to have a hard time just walking around our lawn the next.

I was feeling a little anxious, but not alarmed. My five years' training was operating. I don't like to see women hovering over their men, telling them what to eat, not to take a drink. I never wanted to play the role of nursemaid and I don't much like to see other women do it either. I admit I like to think of my man as not only able to take care of himself, but able to take care of me too when necessary. Maybe I had overprotected myself against alarm, but I went to sleep that Friday night confident that after a good night's sleep, settled in our own winter home and with no more driving to face, Limey would wake up feeling fine.

He did not.

"I feel lousy," he said the next morning. "Stay in bed and rest," I urged, but Limey hated lying in bed. It soon became apparent, however, that he needed help in getting dressed—especially in arranging his shirt, so that in his spatial confusion he did not put it on backward. But he ate his breakfast, a rather hearty one, despite some difficulty in getting his cup of coffee up to his mouth without spilling it. "I'll be okay," he assured me. "Don't worry." But his face looked gloomy.

Our Sarasota friend, who had thoughtfully stocked the

refrigerator with our breakfast needs, appeared a little later in the morning to take me marketing. Limey was very fond of Hannah and seemed more himself when she was there. Limey usually perked up quickly when someone he really liked came around, and I was relieved to see his depressed mood lighten.

I stocked up on staples and bought food for a few days and a supply of bourbon, scotch, vodka, and some wine. After lunch we all rested for a while and then Limey and I went to meet Hannah and her husband for a walk on the beach.

It was what we called at the Cape a "beachy" day. Some clouds, a little wind, and just enough sun—not so bright it bothered Limey, but enough to be pleasant. The salt water smelled good. It was an important walk, one to remember. The four of us started off together, and then Matthew and I walked ahead and Limey followed slowly with Hannah. Along the way he picked up a couple of small, perfectly shaped shells delicately shaded gray and amber; they are still intact on a shelf above his desk. Limey looked well on the beach in his dark blue turtle-necked shirt, blue cotton slacks, sneakers, and dark sunglasses that made him look as if he belonged either to Hollywood or the Mafia. It was a happy afternoon: exactly what I had been aching for those December and early January weeks in Connecticut when the car had been too cold, the weather gloomy, the oil bill too high, and our anxieties depressing. It was going to be a fine winter.

We parted cheerfully, Limey and I happy that we were

there, delighted with all of Hannah's plans: tickets for the opera on Monday night, a visit to the Barnum & Bailey museum planned, tickets for a jazz concert the following week, an outing to a special restaurant on the water. "And go to the fish restaurant tonight," Hannah said. "You'll like it, and we'll see you for dinner tomorrow night with friends we want you to meet."

When we got back, Bob had returned from his own exploring of the Key, and we sat outside with our drinks. "You sure you want to go out for dinner?" I asked Limey. "I can fix something here."

"No, I'd like to go to the fish place Hannah talked about. I'm all right." He did seem okay, except that he complained of feeling cold although Bob and I were comfortable. When we moved indoors, Limey was still cold and I turned on the heat.

Around eight or eight-thirty we went in search of the fish restaurant. The place was quite crowded and Limey was not good at standing for a long time, but he leaned against a wall and we didn't have to wait more than five or ten minutes. The maître d' was leading us to a table, Bob in front and I beside Limey, when suddenly Limey's knees buckled under him and he would have fallen down if a man on the other side of him had not grabbed him quickly. I could not hold him up alone. Limey was upset by the incident. "Ridiculous thing to do," he muttered. "Can't even walk straight."

However, he ordered a favorite fish of his, red snapper, and seemed to enjoy his meal, although he again looked very tired. When we got home he got right into bed, still complaining of feeling cold. I put extra blankets on him, but that didn't please him, as he disliked a lot of weight on his body.

Sunday morning I had to face the hard truth: Limey was not himself, he was not well. I had to give up my fantasy that sunshine and rest were all that he needed. He was decidedly unsteady in walking, he did not want to get dressed (which was unheard of for Limey), and when he sat down for breakfast in a bathrobe he could not manipulate his utensils. He had never been this way before. Bob, Limey, and I had a quick conference and promptly agreed that I should call Dr. Wolf in New York.

As I think back on it now, I realize I felt peculiarly calm that morning. As if for the past few days I had been in a play that I knew, inevitably, was going to reach a climax and that I simply had to let run its course. I know now that nothing we could have done would have made any difference anyway. I am not a fatalist. Neither Limey nor I ever believed that poverty, wars, or even great disasters were the will of God. We believed that man should and does have some control over his destiny, and we are not Christian Scientists. So it wasn't that I thought that whatever was happening to Limey had to happen. But even for the best of diagnosticians there is in the early stages of many illnesses a waiting period during which no one knows what is going to develop. And the popular concept that a stroke is an instantaneous happening is not true. There are many kinds of strokes and the processes can differ considerably. Also at the time I remembered

Limey's previous fluctuations: when he had been tired, or depressed, he retrogressed, as most of us do, and when he was rested and cheerful he was able to do many things he thought impossible.

Fortunately I was able to get Toby on the phone, and after I explained Limey's problems to him as best I could, he said, "I don't happen to know any doctor in Sarasota to send you to. The best thing would be to put him on a plane and send him up here. I want to run him through some tests. I'm sure there's not a bed available, but I'll get one somehow. How will he get to the hospital from the airport?"

"I'll have someone meet him. I'll start driving up as soon as we put him on the plane. Thank God Bob is here to drive with me."

"You'd better arrange to have a wheelchair at Kennedy," Dr. Wolf said.

The word "wheelchair" hit me hard. I was sitting in Mrs. Vogel's small office (we had no phone in our apartment) and I could look out at her very green lawn and small flower garden. I had a strange feeling then that I was going to have again and again: of course I knew that this was going to happen (as if I had read the script someplace), and yet I didn't believe that it was happening. It was preposterous that we should turn around and go back North when we had only arrived the day before yesterday. We were not jet-setters who spent our weekends in Florida. But who were we? I felt trapped by stereotypes, sad-looking people on the six o'clock news: middle-aged, sick, wheelchairs, in a strange place where we had no connections, confused about what to do. The telephone conversation had been so fast, a decision made so quickly. Months of planning swept away—was it the right thing to do because Toby Wolf had said so?

I believe I cast my die then and there, although not consciously. After my initial shock I was relieved that someone else had made a decision. Toby Wolf was a good doctor, he knew Limey, and because he was a friend of long standing he had to be personally involved—he was going to run the show. It was a decision I never regretted, although, as it later turned out, he was not to be the only director.

Making plans cheered us all up in an odd way. Limey said he wasn't sorry to get the hell out of Florida, he was freezing. Bob had made a Monday-morning plane reservation for himself and now offered to turn it over to Limey and drive the car back. "You can fly up with Limey," Bob said. "I don't mind bringing the car back."

"Hila doesn't fly," Limey said.

If I had been a nobler wife that would have been the moment for me to make the grand gesture, but all I did was to nod agreement with Limey and be grateful that Bob was going to drive back North with me. I did not think that was a propitious moment to tangle with my own complicated problems about flying. The last thing Limey needed was a panicky wife; nor was I about to expose myself to any extra anxiety. I found that as Limey's illness presented more and more problems I had to learn to deal with the essentials as best I could and try my damnedest not to be diverted into stomach-churning side issues. To be the noble, self-sacrificing little woman was a charming image but one that I could ill afford to indulge in. Actually that role had never attracted me, but I had a strong premonition that I was now going to have to lace up my stays and be a Woman Who Can Take Responsibility. I only hoped I would have the grace not to grit my teeth about it.

I called our two sons, one with his wife and family of five children near Hartford, Connecticut, and the other with his wife and one baby in Cambridge, Massachusetts, and gave them our sad news. Jimmy, our younger son in Cambridge, said that he wanted to meet his father at the airport and take him to the hospital, so that was arranged.

My next job, and one which I dreaded, was to tell the couple who owned the motel that we had to leave. We had definitely taken the apartment for twelve weeks, and now after three days we had to go, and this was, of course, their choice season: the rest of January and February and March. "Christ, if we were rich I'd be glad to pay them for the whole time, but we haven't got that kind of money," I was muttering half to myself. Limey was lying on the sofa and Bob and I were sitting at the dining table.

"You'll probably have to pay them for at least a month," Limey said.

"Maybe you can get away with a couple of weeks," Bob offered.

I saw Mrs. Vogel outside in a bright pink smock, and she waved pleasantly to us through the window. "I guess

I'd better get it over with," I said, and went out to talk to her.

"My husband is sick," I said. "That's why I had to use the phone in your office, but I made all the long-distance calls on my credit card. I don't know what to say about the apartment. I feel awful about it, we all do, but I have to put him on a plane in the morning and he's going into the hospital . . ."

"I'm so sorry," Mrs. Vogel said sympathetically. "Do you need anything? Is there anything we can do?"

"I don't think so. There's nothing to do. I want to get straightened out with you about the apartment . . ."

I followed her into the office. "Let's see, you came here Friday night, and you're leaving Monday morning . . . that's three nights. So you owe me for three nights. I'll take it off your deposit, and give you a check for the balance."

I was stunned. "You keep the deposit. That's the least that's coming to you."

"You were here three nights, that's what you pay for," she said firmly.

I did not want her check, but she was so insistent I felt that I would be insulting this remarkable woman if I persisted in offering to pay her for more time than we had spent there. I was even hesitant and shy about offering her the refrigeratorful of food I had bought, but she accepted that graciously.

I came back to our apartment feeling quite light-hearted; not only because we weren't going to be out a large sum of money but because people are decent, and when you are in trouble, strangers can be very kind. I believe it was Blanche, in Tennessee Williams' *A Street-car Named Desire,* who said, "I always depended on the kindness of strangers." Something to remember.

Limey decided to go back to bed, which worried me, but since he looked as if he might fall asleep I walked over to Hannah's house on a canal a few blocks away. I told them our plans. "Why don't you stay here?" they asked. "There's a fine hospital in Sarasota, and we have friends who can recommend a doctor." They were soft-spoken, not insistent, which I appreciated, and the sunshine and beach were tempting. The thought of packing up again and driving back to New York the next day was far from attractive. But my instinct said no. We had chosen Dr. Wolf, and we should stick to our decision. Time after time I would have to deal with people who tried to impose their advice. I had to learn to say, "Thank you very much," and go my own way. As long as I trusted Dr. Wolf, I was not going to shop around for medical advice (which is not to say I was opposed to consultation) from other doctors or from friends.

I remember that when I was pregnant I suddenly seemed to meet no one but pregnant women, and each of them had a different experience and different advice to give. The same is true of illness: no matter what you have, suddenly everyone either had it or has a cousin who had it and will tell you what to do. It's hard to ignore all these well-wishing friends and acquaintances, especially when you are upset and want confirmation that you *are* doing the right thing. But while I do not believe any doctor is infallible, you have to either have confidence in your doctor or get rid of him; to let yourself be confused by what happened to so-and-so and what his doctor said can be the path of disaster.

I have found that in dealing with any professionals, and especially those in medicine, one must not be afraid to ask questions and demand answers, but to understand at the same time that even the best do not know all the answers. One thing I do want from a doctor is his undivided attention when I am talking to him; I can't stand a doctor who keeps looking at something on his desk or talking on the telephone when I am in his office trying to have a discussion with him.

When I came back, Limey was dozing, but he opened his eyes long enough for me to tell him that I was going for a short walk on the beach with Bob. "Go ahead, I'll be asleep anyway," Limey said.

It was a lovely day, less windy than the day before, and warmer. Bob and I walked along the beach drinking in the marvelous salt air. We spoke very little; I was trying hard not to think, making every effort to give my mind over to my physical surroundings, the sand, the shells, the sea, and the sky. Bob and I had driven a short distance to a part of the beach where there were no houses, only sand between the Gulf and the lagoons. It was beautiful, so much so that I said to Bob, "I'm going to drive back and see if Limey feels up to sitting out here for a while. He will love this."

Limey was awake, and he did want to drive to the

beach. I parked as close as I could so Limey would not have to walk much, and he was soon sitting on a log on the sand. Bob was nowhere in sight.

My spirits rose. Nothing really awful had happened, I told myself: Limey had a retrogression and maybe that was a common pattern; after a week or two in the hospital we could come back to Florida if we wanted. Limey looked good on the beach. He loved looking at the water, and I loved looking at him against that background. But Limey wasn't comfortable sitting that way for long, and when he tried to get up, he couldn't. He could not pull himself up and I was not strong enough to support him. I tugged and he tried, but we could not get him to a standing position.

"Where's Bob?" Limey asked.

"He must have walked down the beach." There was not a soul in sight.

"I guess I'm a lump on a log," Limey said morosely, and we both giggled.

"This is ridiculous," I said determinedly, and we tried again to get him up on his long legs. Limey was not a heavy man, but he was absolutely dead weight. I pulled and he tried and we were both laughing, with a tinge of hysterical desperation, at the absurdity. Finally I spotted a sturdy young man coming down the beach, and I promptly hailed him, and he got Limey to his feet. Together we helped him to the car. Then we really laughed.

Limey insisted that there was no reason not to go to Hannah's for dinner, and so we all went as planned. Once Limey was sitting down he was fine, except for

needing help with his food. His speech and his mind were
as sharp and clear as ever, and as I look back, I am grateful that we had that pleasant and stimulating evening.

   We had asked for a wheelchair at the Sarasota airport
and Limey sat in it while I picked up the reservation. It
was Monday morning and the place was filled with ex-
pensively tailored, well-tanned businessmen, carrying
their leather attaché cases, probably weekend commuters
from New York. You caught phrases about so-and-so's
boat, yesterday's tennis game, a board meeting and the
stock market—and I hated every one of those men. They
looked so healthy and *active*. Limey, who had usually
been taken for ten years younger than he was, now, in the
wheelchair, looked his age. I experienced my first feeling
of our being set apart. As if someone had tapped us on the
shoulder and told us, "You're on the other side now, kids,
you don't belong with the healthy, beautiful people anymore, you've got an unpleasant blight."
   Damn the beautiful people. Limey, in his jaunty Brooks
Brothers hat, was better-looking than any of them, and I
knew he was smarter. Franklin Delano Roosevelt had run
the country from a wheelchair and we haven't had anyone to match him since. I was glad I had on my chic
black Bergdorf Goodman pants suit and my extrava-
gantly expensive boots, and I wallowed in the special
attention the airline attendants gave us. Limey was
wheeled through the doors first, before any of those
bronzed, impatient men on line, and I was able to board

the empty plane with him and see that he was comfortably settled. We had a cheerful parting, with a lover's kiss.

Bob and I watched the plane take off, and I guess my emotions showed, because Bob suggested a drink before leaving. It was a good thing to do. Then we took off.

It was a bizarre trip. Ironically I was in the very position where at times during the thirty years of my marriage I had fancied myself: on the road, away from home with all its demands, with an attractive man whom I liked very much. To be with Bob was comforting. He was a good companion, amusing, like Limey interested in his surroundings, in good food, and a steady, excellent driver. Monday evening I called Dr. Wolf from the motel where we stopped. He gave me good news. "Limey's in the hospital, he's in good spirits, and things don't look so bad. He's better than I expected, although it was wise to send him up here. Jimmy's with him, he walked up and down the corridor with Jimmy and he had a pretty good supper. Call me up tomorrow afternoon at the office and I'll have the results of some of the tests. I feel more encouraged than when you called me on Sunday."

I was ecstatic, and we celebrated with an excellent dinner. Knowing how anxious I was to get up to New York in a hurry, Bob said, "Wake me up whenever you get up, no matter how early. Call me on the phone."

I woke up around six, and picked up the phone next to my bed. "Please call Mr. Graham in Room 109 and tell him it's time to get up." There was a dead silence for a few seconds. Then a male voice said, "I'll ring the room, *you* tell him to get up." It was funny, but alone in my room I got a fit of giggles out of proportion to the humor, and I realized how close to the edge I had been operating. Tears could have come just as easily.

We did make an early start, and around two o'clock in the afternoon, when I felt sure Dr. Wolf would be in his office, we stopped to telephone. We had left the highway and were traveling east to get to the Chesapeake Bay Bridge because Bob had figured out we could save time that way. The day was sunny and warm, and we were on a secondary road that wound its way through gentle, sweet-smelling farm country. It was hard to believe that there was snow in New York, and dressed only in jeans and an open shirt, with bare feet, I could have been on a picnic in the country. I quieted the pangs of anxiety that popped up by going over Dr. Wolf's words in my mind. He had said it didn't look serious, he had said he was encouraged—Limey was going to be all right, and at some later date we would both laugh about this crazy trip to Florida. Limey would say he hadn't wanted to go there in the first place, and I would nod and say, "Of course, darling, I should always listen to you"—both of us knowing that that was a big family joke.

Bob pulled into a dinky gas station—not one of those big, flashy places you see on the highway—and while he was getting gas I sat in a glass telephone booth close to the road and dialed New York. Toby Wolf came on the phone quickly. "Limey had a massive stroke sometime this morning. His left side is paralyzed and his right side is not very good. I am so sorry . . ." His voice trailed off.

"His whole left side?"

"Yes."

"Can he talk?"

"Yes, he can talk. There's not much to do now except wait and see. When will you get here?"

"As fast as I can. I hope tomorrow. I'll call you tonight. Do you mind?"

"Of course not."

"How is his mind?"

"He seems alert. I'm sorry, Hila, I wish I didn't have this news for you."

"I know."

I sat in the phone booth without moving. I didn't cry, I'm not sure I felt anything except a heavy, heavy weight. The sun was still shining, the countryside was still calm and lovely. I don't know how long I sat there, seconds, minutes . . . I didn't know what town I was in, not even what state, but I remember the quiet, the blacktop road, watching a tan pickup truck go by, hearing some young children playing around the garage. That place, whose name I do not know, has been printed indelibly on my mind. Finally I got out of the phone booth and called Bob. I told him the news.

My shock was reflected in his face, and then I sobbed. He put his arms around me and held me close to his nice teddy-bear body. We didn't talk much when we continued our driving, although we both felt a greater sense of urgency. Thank God Bob didn't feed me any of the clichés or syrupy talk I was to hear later on. After a while I learned not to listen, but I don't think I could have taken it then—the Pollyanna talk about how Limey was going to be all right because so-and-so had had a stroke and was now riding a bike, or so-and-so couldn't walk and was out dancing every night—and "it could be worse." How I got to hate that phrase "it could be worse." What could be worse? Was I supposed to receive comfort from the fact that other people had worse strokes, less money, inadequate medical care, no love? I am perfectly capable of compassion for those less fortunate than I, but for God's sake I did not want their sufferings offered to me like a compensating consolation prize for our own tough luck. I had my own serious problems to cope with and I did not appreciate being plied with the sufferings of the world at that time.

What I did want, and got from many friends, Bob gave me on that trip: warmth, affection, and most important of all, I now realize, he remained the same in his attitude toward me. There was absolutely no change in our relationship. He did not look at me with sorrowful eyes, nor did he make me feel that I had been singled out for TROUBLE. We talked as we always had, about everything, about nothing. He allowed me to feel normal, at ease, to laugh at his witticisms, to make some of my own. If we talked about Limey he didn't put on a funereal voice, and I was able to enjoy the dramatic beauty of the Chesapeake Bay Bridge, the magnificent ride across that span of water with no land in sight. It seems to me that when people are in trouble they do not need a sign hung on them that spells out TROUBLE, a sign that obliterates all else. They need to be kept in contact with a real and total world, their everyday landscape, of which their trouble is only a part.

When I called up Toby Wolf on Tuesday evening there was no change. We made the trip back much faster than we had going down. I remember reading signs along the highway—LAST EXIT—the words were ominous and added illogically to my gloom. I think we had left Sarasota around one o'clock on Monday and were driving up Park Avenue by two o'clock Wednesday afternoon. Our arrival in New York had its light side. I found myself involved with, and comically dense about, making practical decisions. What to do about the car? I went through a lengthy, boring conversation with Bob over whether I should drop him at the bus terminal or Grand Central Station, or did he want to stay on in New York? Should I take him to a friend's house? . . . It went on like an old Mike Nichols–Elaine May routine until, waiting for a green light, I suddenly said, "My God, what are we talking about? You take the car and go wherever you want and take it up to Connecticut with you. I don't want it in New York."

Then there was the problem of where to stay. I had the choice of Dr. and Mrs. Wolf's apartment, a few blocks from the hospital, or my cousin Pat's, also a few blocks from the hospital. They were all being enormously kind, but maneuvering myself around that ridiculous problem of not wanting to hurt anyone's feelings (as if where I stayed really mattered) assured me I was sleepwalking. None of it was real. I stayed at my cousin Pat's, and it is to her monumental credit that our close friendship withstood the trial of a house guest who monopolized the phone (people kept calling constantly to find out how Limey was and wanting to be called back), whose emotional temperature fluctuated from minute to minute, and who was prone to flooding the house with tears at odd moments.

No sooner did I arrive at Pat's ample apartment on Fifth Avenue, and open my suitcases in the bedroom vacated by her son at college, than another problem presented itself. I had nothing but summer clothes to wear and New York was very cold. It all seemed ridiculous with Limey lying paralyzed a few blocks away. Two things seem to happen in a personal crisis, at least for me: small problems become an emotional trauma on one level and totally insignificant on another. I couldn't have cared less about what I wore, and yet I felt idiotic tears roll down my cheeks as I looked at my bagful of white slacks, cotton dresses, and bathing suits. I was crying not only because Limey and I were here instead of there but because I felt stupid, unable to think what to do about it.

"You expect too much of yourself," Pat said. "You expect to react perfectly normally when your life right now is not normal. You've had a bad blow."

I must remember that, I thought. I was supposed to be a strong woman, and I wasn't used to this kind of slow motion of my brain and my reactions, like learning to swim underwater. Pat, who is considerably taller than I, fixed me up with some jeans and a heavy coat belonging to her thirteen-year-old son. Later I telephoned Bob's wife in Connecticut, and she generously went into our cold, closed-up house, packed up a bag of winter clothes for me, and had them delivered via another friend to Pat's apartment. The kindness of friends is even more dependable than the kindness of strangers.

I was aching to get to the hospital to see Limey, and I was terrified. Even with a warm coat the air felt icy and the few blocks' walk to the hospital was an ordeal. Laughing children were coming home from school and chatting mothers were wheeling baby carriages as if nothing had happened; they had no idea that the small, dark woman hurrying past them had a heart thumping with fear of what she was about to face. Totally paralyzed . . .

Limey was in a room with three other men, flat on his back, pale and drawn, his mouth a little twisted out of shape, and being fed through a tube. I thought he was surely dying. He could hardly speak and when he did his voice was a low, hoarse whisper. I bent to kiss him, and his blue eyes looked at me with love and desolation. There was nothing for me to say to him. He didn't ask me anything about how I got there, about the trip, and I could see that he was in a solitary place of awesome despair that I could not reach. The only thing I could do was to sit and hold his hand and tell him that I loved him and to wish that some of my strength could pour into his stricken body.

Out in the hall Dr. Wolf had little to tell me. I remember saying to him, "If he's going to be a vegetable, please
don't save him." Toby shook his head. "We can't talk
about that now—and his mind is okay."

Limey's mind . . . by general standards, Limey was
not a "smart" man. He never made a lot of money; he
didn't finish high school and he never went to college. He
wasn't interested in money and he had little respect for
institutions of any kind: educational, religious, medical,
or political. Yet he was one of the best-educated persons I
have ever known. When he left home in his teens he
worked as a reporter for various newspapers, he picked
fruit in California, and he worked in lumber mills in the
Northwest. In 1931 he published a novel, *Lumber,* a
tragic proletarian story about the mills. The book was
very well received by the critics, and Little, Brown, his
Boston publisher, wanted him to write another, but he
never did. Some of his stories were published in maga-
zines of the day, and he made a good living for a few
years translating books, including Zola's *The Human
Beast,* from the French. In the late twenties, or early thir-
ties, he became involved with the miners' poverty and
problems in Harlan County, Kentucky. That was a turning point in his life.

From that time on Limey became a defender of civil
rights, and through the ILD (International Labor De-
fense) he worked on the cases of the Scottsboro Boys,
Angelo Hearndon, and others, and became a close companion of the staunch congressman from New York's
Harlem district, Vito Marcantonio, and the civil rights

lawyer Carol King. He also found a loyal friend in Dash-
iell Hammett, a board member of the ILD and the distin-
guished writer who chose to go to jail rather than furnish
a list of names to the House Un-American Activities
Committee.

When I saw him in that hospital room I thought of all
those bound notebooks of manuscript back home that he
had been working on since the time of his first stroke.
None of it was finished—it was all notes and rough drafts
—and it was unlikely that there was anyone else around
who could document the unpublished history of the
political prisoners in the United States, those who were
defended by the lawyers of the ILD, the cases won and
lost. And I had a sad feeling Limey was never going to do
it now.

I walked down the dreary hospital corridor to the elevator trying to think some great philosophical thought
about writing and life, that in a hundred years none of it
would make any difference anyway, but all I could think
of was how awful it must be not to be able to move an
inch by yourself. Was it better to have a mind?

So there I was in New York, a place I had often longed
to be for a month or two in the winter. But not that way.
New York was there with all its vibrant excitement, but I
felt outside of its movement. In the beginning I paid no
attention to it. Central Park, Fifth Avenue, the shops on
Madison Avenue, were there all around me, but I was
living in one overheated, anxiety-ridden room of a big

hospital. It was an all-day vigil with other wives, sisters, in-laws, doing the same thing. We all got to know each other well, the way people do when joined together by the accident of a common critical experience. I was glad that Limey was not in a private room. Here, there was activity, conversation, jokes, and the patients and their relatives cared about each other.

The other men who came and went during the five or six weeks Limey was there were all neurological patients. I remember Mr. Duda, a man around fifty, who traveled back and forth in time, sometimes he was twenty years old (the age of one of his sons), sometimes he thought he was sixty-five. He kept saying that no one cared about him, although his family was clearly devoted. He tele-phoned his wife many times during the day when he knew she was at work and certainly having a rough time trying to hold down her job. Sam was the black male private nurse who took care of Mr. Duda from 8 A.M. to 4 P.M., when a very beautiful, jazzy-looking young black woman came on for the next shift. Limey was crazy about Sam, and for good reason. When Limey wanted or needed anything, Sam knew it and either took care of it himself or called a floor nurse to do it. He never neglected his own patient, although it was silently understood be-tween us that what he did was to be off the record. Sam kept saying to me, "Your man's going to be all right. He knows where he's at, he'll be okay."

There was old Mr. Murray, in the bed next to Limey's. He had a large family, and many of them were at his bedside all day long. But the minute they left, he would try to get out of bed, and sometimes he succeeded and fell on the floor. One day we all heard his doctor explain to him how they were going to give him a cerebral angiogram, which meant running a fluid through his brain. His doctor spoke in a loud voice although Mr. Murray could hear perfectly, and enumerated all the possible side effects: dizziness, nausea, weakness . . . "There can be considerable discomfort, and I must tell you there have been some rare cases of fatality." Doctors never use the word "death." Mr. Murray thought for several minutes while the rest of us held our breath. "Well, I guess I'll take my chances. I sure don't want to go on this way." The doctor went on explaining, as if he had to finish a prepared speech. But Mr. Murray had made up his mind. It was an anxious day when they took Mr. Murray to the X-ray room for his test. He went down sometime in the morning and when he hadn't returned by the middle of the afternoon we were all fidgety. No one talked much. His wife, a large, brown, normally cheerful woman, sat stoically silent. Finally he was brought back to the room in a rage. "The goddamned machine was broken after they put me through that rigmarole. If they think they're going to do that again, they're crazy. Never, never." His wife wept in my arms.

Limey's remarkable mind brought him, and me by association, a special regard and respect in that hospital room. I don't know how they knew—there he was flat on his back, speaking almost in whispers, hardly able to move—but I was told over and over again what a brilliant man my husband was. He seemed to know everything

about the other people in the room; he knew the names of
each of the ever-changing shifts of nurses and had quickly
formed his likes and dislikes, and he had his jokes with
some of them. He was aware of everything that went on
around him, not disoriented as to who he was or where he
was.

In an objective sense, the impact of Limey's alertness
was fascinating to me. The professional staff—interns,
residents, nurses, the top neurologist of the hospital (who
was called in as consultant)—people one so often thinks
of as close-mouthed automatons, were reacting in a *human* way to a brain. Or maybe I am all wrong, maybe
precisely because they were all professionals dealing with
the workings of the brain, they were reacting as professionals. But they seemed to be pulling for Limey in a
special way. For instance, after examining a disoriented
patient in the room, the top neurologist came over to
Limey's bed and shot him some of those strange questions
neurologists seem to favor. "Who is the President?"
"What does 'A rolling stone gathers no moss' mean to
you?" "What day of the week is it?" "What month?" "If
I had sixty-five nickels and spent seven and gave my son
eighteen, and made two telephone calls, how much
money would I have left?" "What's the name of the place
you're now in?" The questions always made me nervous,
and I knew I would have fumbled them. Limey thought
them asinine and the doctors who asked them patroniz-
ing, but with a bored expression on his face he always
came up with the right answers. Except for one: "In my
entire life," he said, "I never knew the day of the week

without looking at the *New York Times*. I don't care about the day of the week, it interests me not at all." The big-shot doctor looked at him with satisfaction. "This man has a mind," the doctor said. "He'll make it." The doctor had an expression of pride on his face, as if he had invented Limey's mind.

But Limey's mind was not the same as it had been, and I knew it, although I could never say it out loud to anyone, even to our sons. He had to have suffered some brain damage, and he did. The damage to the part of his brain that controlled the use of his arms and his legs and his ability to sit up (he could not hold himself in a sitting position alone for a second) was obvious. But there was other damage not so constantly apparent, nor so clear-cut. I am not sure, and I doubt whether the doctors are, how much deterioration is a result of the blockage of blood to the brain and how much attributable to emotional and psychological changes. It is probably a mixture of both. But I sensed a psychological change in Limey—in his involvement with his body, in his lack of curiosity and interest in news events. He dwelt a great deal on the past, and talked about his first wife, who had been dead over forty years. As the weeks went by he suffered some confusion and some hallucinations. In the afternoon he sometimes demanded his breakfast. "You had your breakfast and your lunch, your supper will be coming soon," I'd explain. "I want my breakfast, it's the only decent meal here," he'd yell.

A few times he thought he saw people who weren't there. "Jimmy's out in the hall," he said to me, when I knew Jimmy was up in Boston. "Tell Jimmy to come in to see me." Or sometimes he insisted that his brother Morris, of whom he was very fond, was in the waiting room, and Morris was not there. Those incidents were frightening to me, and I think they upset me more than Limey's wasting body. I had to learn to pay no attention, but to talk quickly about something immediate in order to bring him back to reality. "Did you go to therapy today?" or "Alice is making you some vichyssoise, I'll bring it tomorrow. When you come home we'll have to get a blender so I can make all those good soups for you . . ."

"Yes, that's a good idea," Limey would agree. "We could use a blender for a lot of things." He'd have come back to me, and my heart would quiet down.

He was obedient and cooperative to an amazing degree —he wanted to get better. He spoke a great deal about when he would get out of the hospital and come home. "We'll have a fire and a drink in our own little house— and keep Josephine away from the cheese." Josephine was our food-stealing poodle. Yet it was rare that I could have a conversation with him. He was, understandably, so locked into his own physical problems that in spite of his awareness he was not interested in other matters. When I thought of how angry and frustrated he had been by his earlier handicaps, which had been minor compared to this, it seemed impossible for me, or anyone else, to imagine how he felt about the all-encompassing disability he now suffered. The will to move was still there—but to have absolutely no ability to make that move . . . No wonder it was hard to divert or to hold his attention. I would tell him of a conversation or a visit with a former colleague whom he liked, or read him the headlines in the *New York Times* (in the more than thirty years I had known him he had never missed a day with the *Times* unless it was unobtainable, and that always annoyed him), and he would say, "What's my hand doing? My hand's doing something funny," or "Please wipe my eyes." He rarely responded directly to what I, or any other visitor, had to say, and there was one rather painful scene which occurred during a visit from his former boss, a man Limey truly loved. Max had just returned from a trip to Spain and, being in tune with Limey politically, was eager to give him his firsthand knowledge of the upheaval that had taken place there after Generalissimo Franco's death. But Limey didn't want any part of it. He cut Max off every time he opened his mouth with his repeated requests: "Wipe my nose with a Kleenex," "Move my head," "Wipe my eyes," etc., etc. I felt sorry for Max because he was upset by Limey's condition and, I think, in spite of his own good sense, hurt. Both Max and I had a strong feeling that Limey knew exactly what he was doing—it was his way of saying, "You son of a bitch, coming here looking healthy and well to rub my nose in your damned vacation."

Some visits, however, were very successful. Limey liked to have friends come to see him and, as always, his preferences were very clear. My cousin Pat came over often to bring him the delicate French custards she made. Limey loved them and had me take down her recipe. Another couple brought him a radio that didn't interest him at

first but that we later used a great deal. Friends and relatives had to get used to Limey. I could tell that it was a
shock when they first saw him. Not that he looked so
different, more gaunt and thinner (I had a barber come
in to trim his hair and mustache and beard), but unless I
had a chance to talk to them first they were unprepared
for his helplessness and his almost constant and mechanical demand to have his eyes wiped, his head moved, his
pillows shifted. But the people who were able to get past
that, and whose instincts were wise, were able to reach
him, to give him pleasure and, I think, derive gratification themselves. Those friends talked to him about his
writing, about food—they appreciated his contempt for
the hospital diet—and they weren't afraid to talk about
and to listen to his physical problems. Limey was very
knowledgeable about medicine and welcomed any opportunity to show off. I found it crazy to deal with someone
who could do almost nothing for himself—it was a big
day when he picked up a Kleenex by himself and blew
his nose—and ignore it. He needed to talk about himself.
You had to meet Limey in his new world and yet not
forget that he was a person who was a writer, who had
ideas and thoughts, opinions and prejudices. His world
had narrowed considerably, but it was there and he had
to live in it. But solitary as that world had to be, there
were doors to be opened if you thought about it and
looked hard. I suspect this is true of people with many
kinds of illness, and although Limey was never senile, far
from it, I have noticed that the same approach to communication with the aging, or very old, is usually success-

ful. To ask Limey for advice was the greatest gift I could give him. I asked him how to cook a stew, how to marinate raw fish, whom I should ask to do the income-tax return (he had always done it). I leaned on him as much as I could. When I forgot a name, as I sometimes do, I asked him. "What's the name of the village we visited in Mexico last year?" The answer came back promptly: "Zihuatanejo." "I can't remember the name of that wonderful woman who ran the nursery school Jimmy went to." He came up with it right away, and that had been twenty-five years before. I learned not to burden him with tales of my current experiences in that other, outside world—to tell him what movie I had seen, or with whom I'd had lunch, or what I'd shopped for. I stuck to his hospital world and to the close, intimate home life we had enjoyed—to those areas where Limey could speak with authority, could make his contribution.

Believe me, I did not learn this all at once. That first week he was in the hospital I was pretty numb. By nature I am impatient. I have always run into action precipitously, sometimes with harm to myself and discomfort to others. I get wildly irritated by maids who don't show up, promised business calls that come days late, and dry cleaners who shrink my clothes. Yet in a big crisis I can wait. I have waited calmly for children to come out of operating rooms, for divorces to become final, for babies to be born. Even so, I was surprised by my own calmness that week—it was as if the worst thing that could ever happen had happened, everything else was unimportant, and there was little left to fear. Some people are fond of

saying that suffering and tragedy give one strength. I would call that particular bromide small comfort; too many people get broken by pain and seek all kinds of outlets for release—drugs, alcohol, and incoherent fantasies. About the best that can happen is a kind of resigned acceptance, if you want to call that strength. There is not a damned thing one can do about a serious illness except try to get the best medical care possible. Perhaps the worst suffering is the helplessness, the frustration, the need to wait and do nothing.

"What are you going to do? What are you going to do?" Those words still haunt me. Limey had been in the hospital about two weeks, perhaps a few days more. The intravenous feeding had been replaced with a soft diet and he was getting physical therapy regularly. Every day from Monday through Friday he was lifted into a wheelchair by two attendants and taken to the gym. "Going to the gym" sounded awfully good to me, and I loved to repeat the phrase often, "Limey goes to the gym every day"—as if he were playing squash or punching a bag. I never went to the gym to see what he was doing, I think I knew better, but it was amazing how much fantasy comfort I got from that nice, healthy phrase.

"What are you going to do?" The question was put to me repeatedly as I sat in a dreary restaurant having lunch with a well-dressed, well-preserved, preoccupied couple in their late sixties, close relatives whose lives had always been intertwined with mine. They had come in from out of town for a couple of days to take care of some business and also, they had said, to visit Limey in the hospital.

They were a pair I would naturally count on. Somehow or other, however, they had managed not to get to the hospital to see Limey (staying in town for a later train had seemed unthinkable), and I had come downtown to meet them before they took their midday train back to their country home. "What are you going to do?" The wife looked at me nervously, uncomfortably, and I kept saying, "I don't know . . . I haven't had time to think, and besides I don't know how Limey is going to be."

It was a hurried, edgy lunch. They seemed eager to get away from me and, as the months went by I could only assume that they wanted to, needed to, keep their distance from our tragedy. My thinking must have come close to the mark because that couple, during all the ups and downs of his illness, never came to see Limey or me once, although I told them several times that he had particularly asked for them. They sent expensive gifts of fine scotch and imported pâté, for which I thanked them, but I could never get myself to tell them Limey no longer had any taste for such delicacies. I realized they were trying in their own way to make a thoughtful gesture and the fact that I could not enjoy their gifts much either was my problem, not theirs: I felt like a kid with an F. A. O. Schwarz toy from absentee parents when what was wanted was a warm, close hug.

When I left them that day, however, I thought, not about "what I was going to do," but what I, what Limey and I, had become. Practically overnight we had moved from that comfortable middle-class niche where people got invited to dinner and gave dinner parties, spent their weekends gardening, went to movies and theaters—were essentially very much like their friends—to being a couple set apart. For some people we were going to become an emotional burden they'd rather not have to face.

In my inability to provide a reassuring answer to that insistent question, "What are you going to do?" I was discovering a new side effect to Limey's illness that no doctor could treat and that is not noted in the medical journals. Were we going to be outcasts, pariahs, people who were to be visited, if at all, out of a grim sense of duty or pity? Were we going to be another statistic in someone's research of a middle-class family who lose all their savings, their house, their dignity, in caring for a long-term illness that had no cure? Would our anger eventually turn into a gnawing resentment that would inevitably turn us against each other? All these questions led directly to the crucial one: if Limey were to remain paralyzed, did I want him to live or did I wish that he might die?

At that time I pushed the question from my mind. I was not writing Limey off. Even when friends wept in the hospital corridor, and their eyes said to me, "Hila, how can you bear it?" Limey's life was dear to me and had meaning. He was alive, and that hospital room was the center of my existence. I needed Limey in my way as much as he needed me, and he needed me in a tremendous way. He needed me in a way that no one, not he, not our children, had ever needed me before, and that knowledge had its own headiness. I am not talking about feeling saintly, God forbid, or martyr-like, but rather as if everything I ever had to give to someone was being used, that I was being tapped to my innermost depth, I was hitting on all cylinders at high speed. Limey's needs were forcing me to expand to my utmost potential—I could no longer be what the school jargon calls an "underachiever." And that is an experience, painful and hard as it is, that cleanses away a lot of the garbage one ordinarily carries around. But Limey's pain, my pain, his *need,* did not give me strength as such, unless that can be translated into sharpness, a deeper awareness, an intensity of emotions that one does not come upon when life is running smoothly.

Nor did illness make a hero of Limey—he had little use for heroes. He complained, he cursed (his four-letter words amused some nurses and shocked others), when he wanted his ass wiped he said so, he never used euphemisms, and he cried when he was hurt. He was totally honest with himself. There was no faking anything with Limey and his tearing away of all pretense demanded the same rock-bottom straightforwardness from me, and I am grateful to him for that.

That couple who absented themselves from our lives deprived themselves of sharing any part of that experience with Limey. But our friends, for the most part, were tremendous, and I think those who became closer to us than ever before must have done so because they felt some part of what I have been trying to explain. Limey could still enrich other people's lives, but not, dammit, because he had a special courage, or heroism, or any of the endowments glorified in books about the sick and the handicapped. In his suffering, as in the rest of his life, he never put on an act for anyone: he was blunt, frustrated, opinionated, funny, sometimes rude, uncompromising in many ways, demanding, and lovable.

The improvements that Limey made seemed infinitesimal, yet each was monumental. To go from being fed through a tube to being fed real food ("If you can call this mush real food," Limey said) was a big step; from lying on his back in bed to sitting in a wheelchair was another big one. His left leg and arm were dead weight. He could move his right leg and his right arm and hand, but he could not control his movements. When he sat in the wheelchair his body kept slumping down and he was constantly wanting to be pulled up. His head lurched to one side; several kinds of neck collars were tried but none seemed to help. He could not hold himself up in a sitting position for a second. He hated the wheelchair, was never comfortable in it, and after ten or fifteen minutes screamed to go back to bed. In the hospital they timed him in the wheelchair and kept him in the chair from an hour to two hours a day. "Get me out of this torture," he yelled. His voice had become close to normal with only an occasional slur, yet he insisted that he couldn't talk. "I can't understand myself, so how can anyone else?" he demanded.

Trying to keep him comfortable and to keep him from getting bed sores was a major concern. Considering that he was in a very large hospital, understaffed, as usual, the nurses and aides did a pretty good job. I bought large quantities of talcum powder and body lotions for back rubs. I was there every day, usually in time to feed him his lunch, and stayed until I gave him his supper. I learned about things I'd never heard of before; I had to buy a pair of lamb's-wool pads at the outrageous price of twelve dollars to protect his heels from getting sores, and a lamb's-wool sheet to put under his back. He could not turn himself over in bed and was supposed to be turned from side to side regularly, although that did not always happen, but his skin tone and body were really kept in very good condition. Limey was incontinent and that was something that worried me a great deal. How was I going to handle that at home?

"That may get straightened out," Dr. Wolf told me. "Don't worry about it now."

I learned that with a stroke patient, and I imagine this is true of many other illnesses, a doctor can give no clearcut, definitive prognosis. He cannot say he is going to recover the use of his limbs in four weeks or in eight weeks, or that he will recover at all. This is a very hard problem for relatives and friends to deal with. They want to know. I wanted to know, but I could tell that there was no sense in pushing for answers that were impossible to give. I had to use my own eyes and my own common sense. You keep hoping and you hang on to straws. I have seen families get into a big muddle because of the uncertainty and because each person is listening to what he wants to hear. A doctor can say, for instance, "He may live three weeks or five years." One person hears only the three weeks, while another fastens on the five years. Neither one has really listened to what the doctor said and the ensuing confusion, all the back-and-forth family discussions, the panic that the patient is going to die in three weeks, are no help. You have to listen, to sweat it out day by day, and to believe what your eyes tell you. No doctor is God, nor does he have a crystal ball. A person can come out of a thorough physical checkup with an excellent record and drop dead of a heart attack the next day. There is no blueprint. Watching the course of an illness is a patient, waiting game.

Don't worry about anything in the future now—take each day as it comes. God, if only I could imprint those words on my mind, could make them become part of me, I'd be all right. To project into the future was the path of disaster. "What are you going to do?" was an impossible question, and when it raised its ugly head at four o'clock in the morning I took a couple of pills and willed myself back to sleep, sometimes successfully.

So there I was, writer turned nurse, living each day in the hospital learning to take care of Limey. There is no question in my mind that good nursing care can do more for a patient than any other one thing, which is not to put the doctors down. But a nurse sees a patient throughout the day and night, gets to know him in a way a doctor cannot, and in keeping him comfortable helps his spirits and his outlook, two of the most important factors in the recovery from any illness.

Then one day I was abruptly jolted out of my routine by a handsome young woman friend in Connecticut, a nurse, of whom Limey was very fond. "Are you working?" Lois asked me on the phone.

"Working?" Her voice had sounded accusing. "For God's sake, I'm at the hospital every day. If you mean writing, of course not."

"You have a book due in the spring, haven't you?"

"Yes, I was going to work on it in Florida, but a few things intervened. Listen, Lois . . ."

"You listen. I'm coming down and I'll nurse Limey. Find out if I have to clear with anyone at the hospital to get in as his nurse. I have a place to stay, so that's taken care of. Never mind, I'll call the nurses' registry myself. I'll be there Monday morning."

"Lois, that's fantastic, but I haven't thought anything about money yet, I . . ."

"Shut up, will you. I don't want to hear anything about money. I love Limey, do you understand? I love you too. Goodbye." I wept when I hung up the phone.

On Monday morning Lois, practical nurse in her crisp white uniform, was by Limey's bedside. He adored her, and with good reason. She was full of humor, a little fey, terribly efficient under a deceptively scatter-brained façade, and very good-looking. Exactly right for Limey. She was going to stay until after lunch and I would come over in the middle of the afternoon when Limey woke up from his nap.

That left me in that college boy's zany room (weirdo underground posters staring at me from the walls) with my typewriter, a ream of blank paper, and a lot of blank hours. Work. Goddamn Lois, who needed such a good samaritan? I wondered if I could ever write again. I looked at my notes, I looked out the window, I even slept in the middle of the morning. I didn't want to write. I wanted to be in that hospital room with Limey. I wanted to know what was going on there: Had he eaten his breakfast? Was he going down to the gym? How were his spirits today? Was he in the wheelchair? Was Mr. Levin going home? Was my friend Mrs. Murray there?

Damn, I was letting myself be pushed around like a ninny. Limey was my husband and I should be there with him, taking care of him. Well-meaning Lois had one hell of a nerve pushing me out . . .

I thought about the questions people most frequently asked me: "How do you work? Do you have regular hours for writing? How many hours do you write a day?" And the many letters I got from the young readers of my books inevitably asking the question "Where do you get your ideas from?"

I answer the questions and I answer all the letters, but I am not sure I have ever made it clear enough for anyone to understand. Writing was a compulsion for me—how else could I have written and published some forty-odd books since 1958, and a lot of magazine stories and articles before that? None of it necessarily made me a good writer, but I always had so many things I wanted to say— stories crowded in on me from some small item in a newspaper, from something someone said to me, from my own indignation or enjoyment or conflict, from my life, my experiences, my endless, consuming curiosity about people—what do other people do with all their fantasies? "You are so disciplined," my friends said to me. But it is not discipline, or anything to admire, when you wonder what else you could possibly do with your time, and when if a day or days go by (and that happens) when you have not been writing you feel uneasy, restless, and you miss the sense of yourself alone—perhaps the assertion of your ego?—in your little study with your thoughts and your typewriter.

But that day I was lost. And I was frightened too. If I wasn't going to be able to work, we were going to have not one sick person but two.

I didn't write a word that day. I went over to the hospital after lunch, while Limey was still sleeping. It was a big relief to be there, where I belonged, by my husband's bedside. As I had before, I sat there all afternoon, looked at Limey, spoke to him a little, walked the corridor, went out for a smoke—somehow the hours flew by, and by six or seven o'clock I was exhausted and eager to leave him for the night. The polluted, fume-filled air of Madison Avenue smelled beautiful, and walking the few blocks home to Fifth Avenue I felt some comfort and stimulation from the city getting ready for the night. I liked to see the people on the street hurrying in the cold, some with their brown paper bags of food for dinner, to think of people dressing for parties, going to the theater and concerts, to see boys and girls walking arm in arm—I was reminded of the big world outside of that hospital room and I was glad that it was there.

Pat asked, "Did you get any work done today?" I shook my head. I had to tell her no. "It must be hard to concentrate," she said.

But I realized it was more complicated than that. I was drawn to Limey's bedside as if by a magnet whose pull I couldn't escape—I had to be there to watch every move, to be sure that everything was being done right. It took me a couple of days to figure out that I was dealing with a hang-up I believe common to many wives: we don't want to trust anyone else, we want to be the closest, and we want to be absolutely indispensable. A self-serving process if ever there was one! Yet I cannot write off such feelings as pure hogwash, because they are not. It is true that a wife can understand her sick husband better than strangers, that she can do things for him a nurse cannot, but she need not be, and should not be, exclusive about her role. I now firmly believe that any woman, or man, who can find work to do while a spouse is suffering a long illness takes the wise course. Pay someone else to do the nursing, someone who is not so emotionally involved as you, someone who leaves the job to go back to her own life. Even if you have to settle for someone without a nurse's training you are better off earning the money than taking on the strain and drain of the care. A sick man or woman needs a healthy spouse if he or she has one, some-one who comes to the sickroom fresh, who holds on to contact with the outside world, who can maintain a life outside of that illness, and, on the practical side, who can make some money, because money becomes more and more important, psychologically as well as practically. The ability to work means the ability to maintain some independence—not to be totally consumed by the suffering of someone you love. (At the same time, however, it took some pain and a great deal of self-examination to come to this realization.)

My friend Lois stayed in New York for a week, I wrote a few pages, and before she left to go back to Connecticut, I went to the Metropolitan Museum of Art. There was a big special show of Impressionists and the museum was jammed. I met my friend Mari there on a late rainy morning. That day turned out to be an important one for me.

The paintings were uneven, we thought, but there were enough that were so beautiful we both refused to be jostled by the crowd and stood to look at them as long as we cared. Then in the pouring rain we went to a coffee shop on Madison Avenue for lunch. We talked little about Limey; nor did she ask me, "What are you going to do?" She had wept when she saw Limey. We talked about the paintings, about her husband's new job, about politics; we laughed as we always did when we were together. It was a lunch very much like other lunches we had had in the past, even down to her fussing about her sandwich and sending it back.

When I left Mari I walked in the rain back to the hospital refreshed by the diversion from my problems. And what a godsend that is. You think you don't want to do anything, you don't feel like being social, you think you cannot stop thinking for a minute about that man lying paralyzed, helpless in that hospital room—but YOU CAN. You can be diverted if you give yourself a chance, if your friends are wise and persuasive (and they usually are—they know), and it pays off. On my walk back up-town, I made a decision, and it was a good one.

Now that generous Lois' week was over, why not hire a nurse to be with Limey in the mornings so that I could work on my book? It seems so obvious now, but at the time it involved putting into a direct, simple action all the complicated feelings I had been having during the week Lois was down. We didn't have much money, but I did have the money we would have spent in Florida. The floor nurses were okay, but Limey needed so much attention: he couldn't even press the button for help, he had to be fed, to be cleaned often. I could not with any sense of ease leave him alone on that overworked floor. The decision was important because, as I look back, I see it as the beginning of learning to face the reality of the problem at hand. In a situation like mine you cannot be conservative, you have to take some risks, some gambles, and I was gambling on work being a lifeline for me, and if it was good for me, it had to be good for Limey too. There was no point in saving the money for later—I didn't know what later was going to bring, and right then I needed the help.

When I spoke to Dr. Wolf, I asked him what he thought about my plan.

"It's a good idea," he said, "if you can afford it."

A registered nurse, I soon discovered, was out of the question. He did not need one and besides, the cost would be monumental. I found it enormously depressing to have to think about money. No one in the United States of America should have to worry about money when a catastrophic illness hits. No doctor could give me a prognosis for Limey, but it was clear, without anyone having to tell me, that he was in for a long siege. How long was impossible to know: this was his second stroke, and he could go on this way for months, for years . . . I had to face the fact that it was highly possible that he would never be able to walk again, and that he would be a permanent bed-and-wheelchair invalid.

Like most middle-class people, I suspect, I was brought up to think like the rich when it came to an illness—you spare nothing, you go all out for the very best. When my sister and I were children we were taken to expensive specialists at the drop of a hat, and a good family doctor came to our house if we had a fever. We were well off but far from really wealthy, yet our parents could afford the best health care available. That would no longer be true today. People like us can no longer kid ourselves that we can buy the same care as Mrs. Rockefeller. We cannot. And the poor are, of course, even worse off—they could as well be living in an undeveloped Third World country rather than in the rich United States with all its medical expertise. One doctor put it to me forcefully: "The middle class is stuck; the very rich and the absolutely impoverished are taken care of, but the man in the middle has no place to go." When I think of the poor in rural communities and city ghettos, however, I question how well the impoverished are taken care of.

It would have been easy to pick up a phone and call the nurses' registry and get a nurse. But without unlimited

funds I had to be more resourceful, use up a lot more
energy and a lot more telephone calls to find someone
suitable whom I could afford. I resented bitterly the practical inconveniences and the emotional toll it took to have
to make judgments based on "How much does it cost?" I
did not want to be bothered with figures, to get emotionally upset when dear friends said, "Hila, do you need any
money?" But you learn. You learn to be realistic, to use
your imagination, to make the best use of what there is
and what you've got to spend.

I was lucky. I found Nellie, the daughter of a friend's
housekeeper. Nellie was a soft-spoken young woman with
a family of her own, a practical nurse with an institutional job in the afternoons. She agreed to be with Limey
from eight in the morning until one in the afternoon,
Monday through Friday. She was superb with Limey and
watched over him like a mother hen, and at a price that I
could manage, generous on her part, but I think not
unfair.

So then I became more compulsive than ever about
working—after all, I was paying someone to make it possible. I started to live on two levels, one deeply involved
life with Limey and the other—with the exception of my
work—a kind of sleepwalking, superficial life without
him. One thing about being as ill as Limey was is that
you either go downhill—and, I suppose, die—or you
make small improvements. To witness his holding his
head a little straighter one day than the day before became cause for a small celebration. To have him show

some interest in the news, to have him aware, to hear him say, "Don't cut your hair, I like it this way," made a day bright. And I think no words of love he ever spoke evoked more poignant feeling than now when he said, "I love you—when are we going home?" Each small change became a big event that I wanted to share with sons and friends and that caused me to smile at strangers on the street. But it was not a straight course. Just when you thought he could finally hold his head up straight, the next day it might be bent sideways again.

I spent my afternoons with him, but I stopped just crawling back and forth between the hospital and home. I went to lunches with editors, to dinners with friends, to an occasional movie or play. I made myself remember that I was a person with a life that had to be led, with an identity outside of the wife in a *Magic Mountain* hospital room, a woman who had to, who wanted to, go on living. It was strange and difficult, and there were terrible times of despair when I didn't know where I belonged or whether I could have a life without Limey by my side. But he was there—he was not a vegetable, he was a person with a mind, and as long as that mind functioned I was not alone. Even with his terrible illness, his temporary hallucinations and confusions, he was there to come back to, and where he was, was home.

I thought I had almost achieved an even keel (meaning that my emotional temperature went up and down half a dozen times a day instead of a dozen) when a lawyer friend suggested that I should get power of attorney. Innocently he mentioned possibilities such as "You may have to sell your house . . . you don't know what may arise. Limey can't write, can he?"

I shook my head, my heart dropping down into my stomach. I will never sell our house, I thought to myself—that would kill Limey. But I was persuaded by the lawyer, who kindly had the necessary papers made out and mailed to me, and in a few days I found myself in a ghoulish scene by Limey's bedside. Perhaps I'd seen too many grade-B movies—but that meeting in the hospital room with a notary public (from the hospital), two nurses as witnesses, with the other patients and their families looking on and me guiding Limey's hand to sign those papers, made me feel like a creep forcing my husband to sign papers on his deathbed. The notary public's loud, insistent voice repeating, "You understand what you are doing, Mr. Colman, don't you?" did not help. Limey did understand perfectly, and whatever thoughts he had he kept to himself. I loathed the whole thing.

And no sooner was that ordeal over than a much more serious problem came up. "I am being pushed to get Limey out of the hospital," Dr. Wolf said. "They make me fill out forms every other day justifying his being here—we really are doing very little for him and Medicare will cut off funds."

I was about to be introduced to the diabolic intricacies of Medicare and Medicaid. Medicare is a voluntary health insurance plan, administered by the federal government for everyone on social security, regardless of income, with a minimal payment of a few dollars a month that is taken off the social security checks. In general, Medicare Part A helps pay for medically necessary inpatient hospital care, and, after a hospital stay, for inpatient care in a skilled nursing facility, and for some home nursing care. Part B (Medicare's medical insurance) helps pay doctor bills, some outpatient hospital services, and some home health services. Medicaid is a different matter. Medicaid provides health care for those who are indigent, and in order to be eligible for Medicaid practically all of one's own resources have to be exhausted. When they say "indigent," they mean really without anything!

For people over sixty-five, Medicare, with all its shortcomings, is a tremendous help. To be under sixty-five and without ample private medical insurance can mean nothing short of total financial disaster if one is struck down by a costly illness—and all illness in this country is costly. The big gap in Medicare (and this is hard to understand in their government gobbledygook literature) is that it will pay for care in a hospital or a certified nursing home *only* when the patient is showing improvement *according to their standards*. In other words they will cut off payments for what they consider simply custodial care. And "they" is whatever local office is administering Medicare in any given community. Even if you are in an institution that provides skilled nursing care, and you need help in walking, in getting in and out of bed, in bathing, dressing, eating and taking medicine, but are not receiving other specific treatment, funds will be cut off. This capricious regulation excludes most patients who have a chronic or terminal illness, or who are simply too old to take care of themselves. It is hard to understand the minds of the legislators who invented this cruelty, but there it is, and one day soon the American people had better change it.

But, as I said, as far as it goes, for those over sixty-five (and it should be for everyone), Medicare is essential. When Limey finally did leave the hospital, we had a bill of something like $23,000, but with Medicare covering 80 percent and our Connecticut Blue Cross picking up the difference, we had to pay only about $54, and that was for the telephone. In addition, there were the doctor bills. Besides Dr. Wolf, the neurologist, a consultant was called in, a general medical doctor saw Limey several times, an ophthalmologist examined his eyes, and a dentist had to pull out a tooth. I must say that all the doctors were more than considerate; no one billed us for more than Medicare allowed, and our CMS (Connecticut Medical Service) picked up the 20 percent not paid by Medicare. However, neither the ophthalmologist nor the dentist was covered by any insurance, so their bills, and of course the nursing care, came out of our pocket.

Now Limey's bed was needed, and he had to be discharged. He had improved somewhat since the day of his massive stroke, but after that initial improvement, there was little change. In spite of some earlier assurance that his incontinence would "get straightened out," it had not. "He'll have to go to a nursing home," Dr. Wolf said.

Nursing home! That's where people went to die. The

thought of a nursing home had never entered my head—both Limey and I had thought that when he left the hospital he would go home. "No," Toby said, "he needs nursing care and daily therapy that you can't give him at home. Talk to the social worker in the hospital."

Nursing homes, social workers—I walked down Madison Avenue in a daze. Nothing in my background had prepared me for this. When I was a young adolescent, my mother had died at home attended by doctors and trained nurses. My father, in his seventies, had gone from his hotel to a hospital for a few days and had quietly died there. There had been no need to deal with our new-fangled bureaucracies. I stopped short on the street—what in God's name was I thinking about? Limey wasn't going to die, and yet "nursing homes" and "social workers" spoke to me of that gloomy, dreaded other world where death and poverty lurked together behind a wall of government red tape. A world I never thought that I, we, with our pretty house, our good life, some money in the bank, would ever have to enter.

I dreaded telling Limey when I went back to the hospital. He was in his wheelchair, in that dreary corridor, his beautiful head listing to one side, his right leg impatiently kicking the air. I chose my words carefully. "You're going to be discharged from here soon."

"Good," he said. "When?"

"I don't know. Toby wants you to go to a rehabilitation place . . ."

"I want to go home."

"But you need the physical therapy. It will help you."

"Where will I go?"

"I don't know . . . we'll have to find the right place."

"Whatever you decide," he said. His docility was sad. I was glad to hear him say, "Get a nurse to get me the hell out of this chair. I want to go back to bed."

Later I sat in a small room waiting for the social worker to call me in. The sad-eyed Puerto Rican woman beside me was wiping her eyes and mumbling in Spanish. When I tried to speak to her, she shook her head and indicated that she did not understand English. I did not need her fear to invade me, I had my own. When the social worker appeared, however, I felt a little less like a person with a number instead of a name, a person whom no one would understand. She was young, intelligent-looking, and pleasant.

I told her who I was, about Limey, and that we needed to find a nursing home that had the kind of physical therapy that he needed, and that we could afford. "No one can afford any nursing home," she said.

"What are we supposed to do? What about Medicaid?"

"Do you own a house? Do you have any property? Any savings?"

"Yes, we do own our house, and we do have a few bonds. I'm working—my husband hasn't earned money for the past few years, this is his second stroke."

She shook her head. "Medicaid varies from state to state, and I can't tell you about Connecticut. But it wouldn't be that much different from New York. You'd have to use up everything you have before you'd be eligible for Medicaid."

"Even my earnings? That wouldn't belong to my husband."

"You'd be allowed a hundred ninety-two dollars a month to live on."

We stared at each other. My hopelessness was reflected in her face. "You'll be better off in Connecticut," she said, "where you and your husband are residents. He'll probably get Medicare for a while anyway."

"What do people do?"

She looked at me unsmiling. "You can put what you own in your name, make your husband penniless, and divorce him. A spouse is responsible for a spouse, and that's the only way out. People do that."

I stared at her in disbelief. "You can't mean that. Are you telling me that I should divorce my husband?"

"I am not telling you to do anything. I am suggesting that it is one thing that can be done."

I was too shocked to say anything. "Thank you," I mumbled, and stood up.

"Have a nice day," she said cheerily with her automatic social worker's smile.

I wished I could have felt anger, rage, but it was all too ludicrous—like suddenly having found myself down the rabbit hole with Alice in that curious, upside-down world where big was little and little was big. I couldn't really believe any of it. Was all the world out of step except me? Once again I was walking down Madison Avenue—God, how well I knew those streets by now, every tailor shop,

every newspaper stand, every drugstore, every beauty parlor . . . I saw three Rolls-Royces drive by in a matter of
minutes.

And then I got angry. I wanted to be one of those crazy
ladies who stood on the street corner and yelled, "Goddamn it, they're all a bunch of shits. Fuck them all."

I thought about my father, who had come to this country as a small boy, an immigrant from Eastern Europe
who wanted to kiss the ground of America. He brought
up his daughters to believe that America was the golden
land, the greatest country in the world—he gave us the
finest education, private schools, good colleges, and
charge accounts. We had every reason to believe him.
Finally the tears came. I felt very much alone, and after
all those years, I longed for my mother. Divorce Limey
. . . How dare she!

I was still fuming when I met a friend for coffee later
that day. "That's disgusting," he said. "And they scream
about the people on welfare who don't get married in
order to get more money. Not that I think Limey would
give a damn. But even on the practical side, it's rotten
advice. If you got divorced you'd lose Limey's social security in case . . ."

He didn't have to finish the sentence. In case Limey
died. Damn them. I wasn't even thinking about the social
security, but outside of all the emotional toll, they could
foul a family up with their inhuman regulations, to say
nothing of the diabolic machinations suggested to cir-
cumvent them.

The outrageous suggestion of a divorce had temporarily

diverted me from the main issue: a nursing home. I walked past the luxurious shops on my way back to Pat's house wondering if I would ever again be interested in clothes. All the women I passed looked enormously chic, and on the spur of the moment I went into a beauty parlor, had my hair shampooed and set, and got a manicure. I bought a new eye shadow and was amused that the old bromides worked. I felt better.

That evening I called our daughter-in-law, Wanda. Both the boys and their wives were in close touch with me, and they had all been to see Limey. Wanda was a speech therapist who worked at a couple of nursing homes, and I needed her advice. "There is only one place I would put anyone I love," Wanda said on the phone. She mentioned one of the places where she worked, near to where they lived, outside of Hartford. "It's a beautiful place, and the people are terrific. I hope they can take Limey."

Wanda mailed me their folders, and the pictures and literature confirmed everything she had said. Even Toby thought the place looked right because the therapy and rehabilitation theme was emphasized. We all agreed that I should go up to look at it, and also to take a look at some other places nearer our own home. I hated to be away from Limey for a weekend, but I arranged to have a woman, recommended to me by a nurse in the hospital, stay with him for most of Saturday and Sunday. Pat, who came to see him often anyway, promised to stop by also.

So this is the way it goes, I thought morosely, riding the train up to Connecticut to pick up my car from Bob's house: first you go around looking at nursery schools, then grammar schools, then prep schools, then colleges, somewhere in between you're out looking for a house, and now you end up with a search for a nursing home.

Looking for schools and houses was pleasanter. Nursing homes, I found, seem to attract a certain kind of administrator who considers it lovable to call all patients "dearie" and who has an addiction for nursery language such as "Are we going to take a bath, dearie?" At one place I visited, a large woman sat across a desk from me and told me that my husband might be eligible for Medicare for a few weeks. "Rarely more than five," she said, and then carefully explained the pauperization of Medicaid. And finally she added, "You can divorce him. It's only a technicality, he probably wouldn't even have to know."

"Is that a common practice?"

She shrugged her heavy shoulders. "Some people do that."

Since I had no intention of putting my husband in her care anyway, I was tempted to let her have it. But I was weary and decided not to waste my breath.

Outside I was not cheered by the well-cared-for shrubbery or the view from the substantial buildings. Schools and nursing homes, I concluded, had one thing in common: the physical layout didn't count for much. The attitudes of the staff and the inmates were what had to be examined, and it was easy to cross off a place where the patients were addressed as if they were so many half-witted children.

After scouting a few more homes, none of them impressive, I headed toward Hartford to Wanda's place. I drove up a long driveway to an interesting, contemporary stone structure, built around a central entrance with two long wings on either side. I walked into a large, sun-filled room dominated by a handsome fireplace ablaze with glowing logs and occupied by perhaps half a dozen men and women in wheelchairs, some reading, some dozing, and also a few young faces. Off to one side was a cheerfully decorated dining room. Floor-to-ceiling windows looked out onto an unmanicured woodsy landscape, and I could see several birdhouses, all busily occupied. This was an atmosphere that I liked, not the depressing scene I had come to expect, and I immediately noticed that, unlike those in other nursing homes I had visited, no one here was in robes, everyone was dressed, and I saw no one sitting staring off into space. Those who weren't reading, or dozing, were chatting with each other or with a staff member.

Rather than doing the interviewing, I felt that I was being interviewed by the administrator. He asked me questions in a businesslike manner about Limey's background, his illness, and so forth. He seemed optimistic about admitting Limey, although he warned me that there would be a wait for a bed.

I left there determined to get Limey into this place, although, despite the favorable impression, I myself, from the beginning, did not feel altogether comfortable there. It had a kind of rarefied Wasp aura. After the New York hospital, I missed seeing any black, Puerto Rican, or Se-

mitic faces around, either among the patients or among
the staff, and I suspect that my interviewer had wondered
what a Jewish girl like me was doing married to the son
of a Presbyterian minister, although none of this was rele-
vant to their taking care of Limey.

It was a bitterly cold day as I drove back to our own
small village, and suddenly it hit me all over again:
Limey was going into a nursing home. I had to pull off
the road while an unexpected outpouring of tears clouded
my glasses. These sudden outbursts were becoming a
part of my life—like living with seizures. You went along,
thinking you were on top of the immediate crisis and assuring yourself that it would all work out, when, bang,
you were hit by the big thing itself; the great big tragic
fact, which, in your busyness with practical problems, you
had pushed aside. But there it was, Limey was paralyzed,
maybe would never walk again; Limey was incontinent;
Limey would never again be the man who drank and
cooked and chopped wood and loved and quarreled and
was curious and interested and totally *alive*. He would
never be whole again.

And at that moment I was crying for myself too. Crying for the woman I was losing: he was no longer the
man who could make me feel amusing, witty, charming,
and gay, a woman whose breasts were admired, whose
legs and ankles were called slim and lovely, who was
loved as a man loves a woman. Dammit, I needed Limey
to make *me* feel alive—he would not be there either to
make me feel a bitch, a dumb klutz, to look daggers
when he wanted me to get off the phone, to yell at me, to

take me in his arms and love me, to let me know that every minute of the day someone was there reacting to *my* feelings, as I to his . . . dammit, I needed only one in my audience, the only person in the world to whom I could expose myself without shame or fear, to let me know that I was alive.

Now I was to be a wife with no one to show a new dress to, to share a book with, a wife who went to nursing homes, who had to deal with social workers and Medicare —another spouse responsible for a spouse in a nursing home. Spouse, mouse—a stupid word. I was a woman. I had to hold on to that.

When I walked into the country store, a gathering place for the people in our village, an acquaintance said, "Hila, you look gloomy." The poor woman probably didn't even know anything about Limey, but I turned and yelled at her: "Is that a crime? I feel gloomy."

It is difficult to indulge in feeling gloomy in the determinedly cheerful United States of America. Our highest-paid professionals, after all, are our comedians. Everyone demands that you be cheerful: "Keep your chin up," "Don't get depressed," "Keep smiling" . . . people are allowed to have temper tantrums if the maid doesn't show, or the furnace breaks down, or the car won't start; they can yell and scream and it's okay, but if you have a serious tragedy you're supposed to put on a brave front and not embarrass your friends or make them uncomfortable with your grief.

When I first spoke to a publisher about this book, he said, "I'm afraid it will be depressing." I had no answer for him in his modish, oversized Madison Avenue office. Laughing all the way to the grave was in.

No wonder we don't know how to deal with poverty and sickness and old age and death in this country. No one *wants* to deal with it. Everyone wants to think that everyone is happy and healthy and young. And I was as brainwashed as anyone. I didn't want to inflict my grief on anyone else, I preferred to weep alone—and yet I often longed for a society where sickness and unhappiness were as familiar, as acceptable, as all those foolish smiling faces in the ads, and all the insistent bromides were not taught to us when we were young. Thank God my sons at least were able to say, "Mom, if you feel lousy, you've got a right." And yet I, who should have known better, felt compelled to put on a bright face for my grandchildren. It was stupid, but I was trapped by a convention not easy to break out of. Children cry, why not let them know that grown-ups cry too?

I know a woman who says she cannot bear to be depressed. I laughed when she told me. Who likes to be depressed? Yet I know what she means. She is lucky because she can pull herself out of it. People take pride in never feeling depressed, as if to be so were a sign of weakness. Why is strength, that kind of cheerful strength, like cleanliness, such a virtue?

I went back to Limey and told him about the nursing home, and if he had to go to a nursing home, he said, he wanted to go where Wanda was. He was pleased when I told him that it was the kind of place where the children could come to see him, that it was close to Jonny's home and easy for Jimmy to get to. It would be a drive for me, from our house, but I could always stay with Jonny and Wanda when I felt like it.

Then there was the wait to hear if and when he could be admitted. I came home to Pat's every day hoping for a message from Wanda. Finally, I think after about two or three weeks, the call came. "Bring Limey up on Tuesday."

Going into action was a welcome relief and, I felt, had to be some kind of progress. I called up the chief of our Volunteer Fire Department about getting the ambulance down to take Limey to Connecticut. After a few calls it was all set for Tuesday morning. Then I arranged to have our house opened, the heat and water turned on. Going home without Limey was going to be awful, but I was also eager to get back into my own house.

It all worked. I couldn't believe how smoothly it worked. My bags were packed and sat beside me at the hospital. Limey's bag was packed, and he, still in pajamas, wrapped in blankets, was waiting with me for the ambulance to arrive. I cried with joy when, right on time, I saw the familiar faces of two young men from our village coming down the hall. I wanted to kiss them. In a matter of minutes they expertly transferred Limey from his bed to a stretcher, I said goodbye for the tenth time to the nurses and patients and families in the room, and we were in the handsome, comfortable town ambulance.

I had never ridden in an ambulance before, and as I sat beside Limey, holding his hand, I thought about all the many hundreds of times we had made that drive together: up the West Side Highway, then the Saw Mill

River Parkway, and on to Route 84. Several times Limey asked where we were. When I told him, "Just past Haw-thorne Circle," or "The place we got lost in the fog, re-member?" or "We're going to make the turn to Dan-bury," he would know exactly. "Stay close," Limey said. "Stay close."

It was not a depressing ride. I felt encouraged. Limey was going to a good place, he would get his physical therapy every day, they were going to teach him how to do more things for himself, and, we hoped, regulate his system so that the incontinence might be cured or handled better.

In a few hours Limey was in a bed in his own room. A handsome room, all to himself, and from his bed he could look out through a large floor-to-ceiling set of double windows to the trees beyond. The nurses were kind, and Wanda and her youngest son, little Jon, were there to greet us. That five-year-old running up and down the halls was the happiest sight I'd seen in a long time. Hoo-ray! This wasn't a prison, a place to be dreaded—it couldn't be, with lively little Jonny allowed to run around. Bless Wanda for having him there.

Limey was sleepy and tired, but I stayed with him for a while. Wanda had a plant for him and little Jon had made a picture to put on the wall. "They're very nice," Limey said, "but take them home. I'll have them when I get home." He was wiser than we were—he knew he had to think of this place as only temporary, and at no time did he want anything around him that indicated more than a very short stay. Later I filled out papers in the office and left. A friend had driven up in my car to get me, and I went home.

Home. I dreaded going into that house alone. "Will you be afraid to stay there?" The boys and our friends had asked because our house is in the woods, somewhat isolated. What they thought of as being afraid was not my worry—besides, I had the dog, Jo, a good watchdog, and some neighbors—no, my fears were not about being alone in the house per se, but about being alone without Limey. I was entering new territory: I would not be able to see Limey every day. I had to work, and the drive was about an hour each way. I had to be able to face long days without seeing Limey, and they seemed to stretch ahead endlessly. *Don't project into the future—that is the path of disaster.* Those words again. Limey is in a good place, I told myself, where they will help him to get better. Maybe if I said that to myself enough times I would believe it.

Many friends and relatives called that night to ask how I was, how Limey was, and I finally found the right answer for both of us. "We're hanging in there, we're okay, we're hanging on."

Part Two

Home alone in our own house, I wasn't all that sure I was going to hang on. I'd been naïve enough to believe that I was going to feel better among our own possessions, an accumulation of years. Our own books, my own kitchen, my clothes, my own bed. Lord, but that large, ample bed for two was cold and lonesome for one. I told myself that I had slept in it alone before. There were times when Limey was working that he had spent a few nights during the week in New York, a couple of times during the course of our marriage when he'd been in the hospital for one reason or another. This was just another such time, I insisted when I huddled, sleepless, in my one warm spot in the bed. Useless fantasy. Limey was in a nursing home, Limey was paralyzed, Limey was slipping away from me into some gray area that was neither life nor death.

The evening I came home a friend and neighbor had

dropped in to see me. A woman a good twenty-five years older than I, vigorous and healthy. She always spoke bluntly. "Everyone has to die sometime," she said. "It's better to let a person die."

"No one is keeping Limey alive artificially," I said sharply. "He can improve you know."

She looked dubious. "When I lose my health I want to go."

"Everyone does," I snapped back. But I thought, you don't know, my friend, you don't know. You'll probably fight with everything you've got to hang on. No one knows what he wants when the time comes. I wasn't the one who could be dying and I didn't know. Limey didn't know either. One minute he could say, "This is torture, let me die." And the next he could talk about the spring or the garden and say, "Let's put in more tulips next year. Lots of different colors." He was more fanatic about his diet than when he'd been well. For several years Limey had been a borderline diabetic. He had kept to a mild diet, avoiding sweets, occasionally indulging in ice cream and cake and using an artificial sweetener. But now when someone would bring him a home-baked cake or cookies, never rich, he wouldn't touch it. "It's not good for me," he'd say firmly, although the doctor had said it was okay if he wanted it.

No one wishes a long, torturous illness on himself, yet if there are any small pleasures left, no matter how tiny, life can, I suppose, be worth hanging on to, so long as the mind is conscious and aware. The irony was that when Limey was healthy he had been fond of saying, "What's

so great about being alive?" I believe he truly had a prag-
matic view about life and death—his matter-of-fact philosophy of not expecting life to be one long "happy"
venture ("I don't expect anything," he said) enabled him,
however, to accept with pleasure, and some surprise, the
good things that came his way. He took misfortune in his
stride as a matter of course. Never once in all his illness
did he say, "Why did this have to happen to *me?*"

Limey no doubt would have liked to die swiftly. He
wrote a poem about it not long before we had gone to
Florida, "Of the Good Death."

> There are some things that I must do
> before I feel I am quite through,
> when the inanity
> —multiple indignity
> of senility, inexorably, stealthily,
> unimaginably,
> grabs a-hold.
>
> Then let you, Death
> withhold my breath,
> quickly, kindly,
> beautifully
> (alas, not prettily
> and never daintily)
> Suddenly

"A good death" . . . is there such a thing? I wondered. "Lucky fellow," Limey always said when a contemporary of his died quickly of a heart attack. "That's

the way I want to go." Yet, sitting there alone, in the house we had fashioned together, adding on a room here or another six feet there when the occasion demanded, a house filled with memories of kids laughing, fighting, being sick, having parties—a house that we had bought a week before we got married and that was a diary of our life together—I thought, "He has something to live for, if I can only get him home." I was glad we had the house, glad we had uprooted ourselves from the lives each of us had led in the city, broken away from the impersonal, temporary unease of apartment dwelling. The house had flaws. Limey had to stoop to go through some of the doorways, the floors were cold, and in the summer our beautiful stream, which never ran dry, also contributed to mildew in the closets. But it was enduring, and I knew that if I allowed it, it would help me.

I was changing. Limey's illness was changing my needs, and I think not for the worse. I had always thought myself, and been judged by my friends, a gregarious person. I was social, and had a wide circle of assorted friends, some very close, others less so. Limey and I never belonged to any one clique; we were both catholic in our tastes and liked and were interested in different kinds of people, although there were perhaps half a dozen couples who were more than friends in a social way, people who, if weeks went by and we didn't see each other, were still our "best" friends—people you could call in the middle of the night if you were in trouble. I know that many people believed that I was more social than Limey, but actually that wasn't the case. I was more aggressive about it, I took the initiative, I did the calling and usually answered the telephone ("It's for you, anyway," Limey used to say), and I made the dates. Whatever arguments we had in that department were not about whether we were having too much or too little social life, but that I had to do the arranging. "If you want to see the Gordons, why don't you call them up?" I demanded of Limey.

"What's the point? You keep the social calendar, I'd have to ask you when we could make a date anyway," Limey answered.

"Nuts."

The passive role that Limey played used to get me mad. He loved having dinner parties at home, he enjoyed going to a small party at someone's house or to a restaurant with another couple. And we also both wanted, and needed, lots of evenings at home alone together, but Limey was clever about leaving our social life to me. "You like to do it," he said, "and if I made a date you'd be sure to tell me it was the wrong night."

"You make these damned assumptions," I yelled.

The heart of the matter was that Limey really believed that people did not find him interesting, and while life kept proving otherwise, and in spite of his strong and authoritative personality, he never quite got over the damage done by his harsh, demanding father during his formative years. As for me, it took me a long time to give up fighting for the impossible. I was never going to change Limey, and eventually I learned, the hard way, that it's stupid to measure what each person does in a marriage or partnership. You do what you can do and the

other person does what he can do, and they don't have to
be the same things. If I was doing an okay job with the
social arranging, why not? Limey did things I couldn't
do, like the income tax, at which I would be a terrible
flop.

It was a damned lucky thing I had come to this conclu-
sion before Limey got sick. I honestly believe that this
attitude helped me considerably in taking care of Limey
and our affairs, so that I did not resent what I had to do
for him and for us. Not that I was always graceful about
it. I was not. But I was able, to a better extent than I
would have been earlier in our marriage, to carry this
philosophy over to more fundamental areas than who
should do the telephoning. Limey was helpless and I was
not, so it was reasonable that I take on responsibilities that
had been his before, including getting the damn income
tax done. Each according to his ability.

Once I was home in my own house, I found that I
needed, wanted, to be alone more. Not that I was shun-
ning people. I was extremely grateful for the attention I
was getting, the many telephone calls, the visits, the invi-
tations. My friends were anxious about my being "alone
in the house." But I got replenishment from being alone
—and I realize now (I don't believe I was aware of it
then) I was saving my energies, my strength, for my visits
to Limey, which were the central focus of my being. It
was an unconscious process. I doubt whether anyone real-
izes, while it is happening, the amount of energy that is
used up, both emotionally and physically, no matter how

healthy you are, when someone close, whom you love, is sick. The most destructive thing you can do is to let yourself get worn out and tired. Then everything goes to pieces: you get depressed, morbid thoughts overrun your mind, you cannot cope. For myself, I found that spending time alone was not an indulgence in self-pity. Yes, of course, many times I was sad alone, but there were times I had been sad when Limey was well and home with me. If you are not a cow, being sad is a part of living, and when you have had enough of it you telephone someone, go for a walk, read a book, turn on the television, sew a hem, cook, chop wood, shop—do whatever it is you do to pick up again.

I felt entitled to a certain amount of depression, even of self-pity (my friend Frances said she would allow me five minutes a day, and I asked her if they were cumulative, like sick leave).

Yes, I was depressed my first night home with Limey in the nursing home. Depressed, but not miserable. I was in my own house and I kept reminding myself that Limey was in a good place. I was sure of it the next morning when my daughter-in-law called up and said, "Everyone loves Limey. They are all very dear with him. Bring him some clothes. Wash-and-wear slacks and shirts, and underwear."

"Clothes?" He'd been in hospital gowns and pajama tops for so many weeks I hadn't thought about clothes.

"Yes. They want to get him out of bed and dressed every day."

"Terrific."

There were some tears when I opened the suitcase of his clothes which had remained intact since our trip to Florida—we had packed that together with fun in our minds —but I was really excited about picking out things for him to wear. His newest suntans, his blue shirts which were so becoming, a warm jacket, a sweater, socks, canvas shoes, underwear . . . He had to be getting better if they were going to get him out of bed and dress him every day. I couldn't wait to get in the car and go up to see him.

The drive from our house to the nursing home is a pretty one. I did not have to go on a highway, and I had the choice of several secondary roads, so I was able to vary the trip as the weeks went by. That first time, however, I paid no attention to the landscape, I was simply intent on getting there. As I drew nearer and nearer my stomach started forming into knots, reminding me of other dreaded times: going for job interviews, to see the principal of the boys' prep school, to have my income-tax return audited . . . It was an illogical fear, as if I didn't know what I was going to find. Maybe it was part of the whole anxiety, or a pattern that had been set in motion when I'd come up from Florida and first went to see him in the hospital in New York. I felt terrified of how I would find him, and I never lost that nervous apprehension during all the times I went to visit Limey.

I parked the car and went inside. The same people were sitting in almost exactly the same places they had been in the day before. Did they each have a favorite spot, or were they put there? Or had no one moved in twenty-four hours? One woman looked up at me and smiled, and I smiled back. Then apologetically, self-consciously—who was I to be able to walk so briskly?—I went down the hall to Limey's room. He wasn't there.

Shaken, I ran to the nurse's station. And there he was, his back to me, sitting in a wheelchair in front of a window. The room held some tables and chairs and a television set, and was, I was told, used for patients who did not go to the dining room because they could not feed themselves. There was one other patient in the room, a very old woman with a face that must have once been lovely, her full gray hair stylishly groomed and adorned with ribbons, in a wheelchair as was everyone I saw, picking away with the outstretched fingers of one hand at something that was not there.

How can I describe the first few minutes of my meetings with Limey at the start of each visit? Was it habit, was it a sly trick of the mind, was it my own questionable ability to live in two worlds, my own apart from his nursing-home life? Whatever, I came to him with a memory of warm embraces, of close hugs, of a tearing response in his face after any separation—it used to take us a few minutes even to say "How are you?" because we just held each other close. Now I walked over to him and he hardly looked at me. He kept staring out the window. I bent down and kissed him, but still he kept his blue eyes turned away from mine.

"Can you see the birds?" I asked.

"No," he said coldly. "I think I can see the shape of a tree. Did you bring me clothes? They want to dress me. I don't know why they want to bother."

"Yes, I brought a suitcaseful. Maybe it will make you feel better. Did you have a good night?"

"No. I had a terrible night."

Finally he turned his gaunt, pain-filled face to me. I didn't know how to read it. Did he hate me because I could come and go? Was his hostility aimed only at me or at the whole world? It was difficult to know how much he could see. He was not blind, but he had no peripheral vision and could not see much, although he was able to watch some television if it was placed just right.

"Do you want to watch something on the telly?" I ventured.

"No. I want to go back to bed."

"I'll take you for a walk first."

"If you want."

I wheeled him up and down the long corridors. We passed other patients being wheeled by nurses or orderlies, but no one greeted anyone. And in the big lounge I realized that none of the patients were talking to each other. That first visit must have been unusual. I thought about the conversation I'd had with the Administrator, when I had come to see the place and hoped to get Limey admitted. He had told me about the interesting, professional patients they had, and I told him about Limey's background, his writing, and how much he had to contribute because of his fine mind. What a bunch of malarkey we were handing each other. What a farce—it didn't matter a damn who these people had been. Whatever they were, they weren't that anymore. Each one was wrapped up in his own self, in his own thoughts, in his own problems. And I had a suspicion that the fine physical setup—the brightly colored walls, the spacious rooms, the beautiful outdoors—was as much for the visitors as for the patients.

After a while I found a corridor that ended in wide glass sliding doors that looked out to a grove of white birch trees. I parked the wheelchair, stood close to Limey, and held his hand. We stayed there alone, quietly, and his right hand, which had strength in it, grasped mine tightly. His face softened, and I knew that at last he was saying hello to me, telling me, "I'm glad you're here." I was happy then that he could not see the tears in my eyes.

It took so long each time to get through that initial hostility of Limey's—God, but he was an angry man— that then it was always hard to leave. Once that awful ice was broken I could get glimpses of my Limey, of his dry humor and the sentimentality behind his outward cynicism. He often asked about the dog, Jo, although he used to complain about what a nuisance she was. "Do you walk her in our woods? Across the bridge? I think we should make some more paths." He was the one who used to walk her there so often, and I realized with a stab that that was what he was remembering . . . *walking*.

The nurses did seem to be fond of him. They took very good care of him, so that he did not get any bed sores. But they had a hard time with his incontinence.

Once when I came to see him the nurses were laughing. "What happened?"

One very young aide actually blushed. "Your husband can say some very funny things," she said.

"What did he say now?"

More giggling. Then Limey spoke up from the bed. "I asked them to clean one end of me of the food that I didn't eat, and the other of the food that I *did*." He gave the half-smile that was the closest he could get to a smile those days, amused at how easily shocked the girls were.

I had a discussion with the head nurse. "I thought there were ways of regulating a patient. Someone told me that if you used a suppository every morning, or every other morning, and put him on the bedpan it would work and that would be it."

"It works with some patients, but it doesn't with him. He has a tendency to diarrhea, and he hates the bedpan so much we gave up."

I knew that he hated the bedpan. He howled that it hurt his back. They tried different kinds but nothing worked, so as far as I could figure out they used pads and simply cleaned him up whenever necessary. This was a big worry to me—what would happen when he came home? I had been counting on the professional nurses and the doctor to establish a pattern that we could follow at home.

Home was where I wanted him to be, but not yet. I had great hopes for what they could do for him in this fine place. My sights were not set very high; in fact, they had been considerably lowered. I forgot about his ever being able to walk again. I knew that was out. I was mainly hoping for three things from the physical therapist, the occupational therapist, and the nursing staff: First, that the physical therapist could teach him to be able to sit on the edge of the bed so that one person could pivot him from the bed to the wheelchair, instead of its requiring two people to lift him. And that person could be me, who would be taught how to do it. Second, that the occupational therapist would provide the kind of utensil and dish that would enable him to feed himself, and would teach him how to use them. Third, that the nursing staff would regulate his bowels and get him to use a bedpan.

I thought these were reasonable and practical goals. I was learning what to expect, and—very important, I found—to whom to turn for specific needs. For instance, I had learned by now that no doctor either knew about or cared to get involved with the problem of Limey's bowels. "The nurses know more about that than I do" was, I believe, without exception the answer I got. I also was learning what Limey and I both needed and wanted from the nursing home: simple, practical benefits that would enable me to take care of him at home.

However, at the same time I was very concerned about his mental attitude, and I soon discovered that I was the one who had to keep plugging away at trying to get him involved and interested in living. Even if they had had a professional psychiatrist available, which they did not, I doubt that anyone else could have made much headway with Limey. I say this in all honesty, not because I take any special credit—I am not smarter nor do I know more than the average layman—but I knew Limey, and I cared. After all, I was going to live with the man, so I had as much at stake in keeping his mind alert as he did—perhaps more.

I brought a radio to his bedside and put a sign on it directing the nurse to turn on the news in the morning and at six o'clock in the afternoon. Later the occupational therapist hooked up a control in a small metal box that was on his bed so that he could turn the radio on and off himself. A small thing like that gave him a lot of pleasure. I brought a tape recorder that he could use instead of his beloved typewriter to record his thoughts. At first Limey resisted the tape recorder. "My voice is no good," he said. "I can't even understand myself." But Limey's "no" was a familiar pattern to me and, as he would be the first to say, not without irony, never stopped me. Almost anything new that was presented to Limey (matzoh balls and me may have been the rare exceptions) was first greeted with a "no." Either "I don't like it" or "I can't do it." It was almost like a nervous tic, a kind of automatic reaction. But once that first verbalization was dispensed with, strange creature that he was, he attacked whatever new thing it was, whether cooking mussels or attempting to write for a medical journal (how positive he had been that he could do neither) with a thoroughness and an aim at perfection that put me to shame. So, when he started using the tape recorder, he really used it, and dictated poems, what he thought of the medical profession, of hospitals and nursing homes (not much), and some beautiful essays on nature, food, nostalgic pieces about his mother, his youth and earlier experiences in his life. Kind friends, one a busy award-winning film writer, generously took time out to transcribe the cassettes. As they wisely said, "Limey needs to see something on paper."

I have been reading over these transcripts, and of all the work that went into the writing of this book, this was the hardest part. The revelation of the inner man, even in the poignant poems, was in such dramatic contrast to the broken body I saw daily, and the inconsequential chatter, that I had to stop and think, did I ever truly know this man with whom I had lived for so many years?

At least once a week, and sometimes more, I brought friends with me to visit Limey. The fact that these visits involved an hour's trip each way was a plus in that only those who cared enough offered to come, and he was protected from a lot of visitors he was not interested in seeing. I think that every sick person needs someone well, and close, to control the number of visitors and pick only those who can relate to the patient and be sensitive to the indignity of his illness. And so, with these special friends, we had picnic lunches in his room, we drank wine and thermoses of martinis. And mainly we talked to Limey. His reactions varied, as did those of the visitors. You had to be able to take Limey as he was, and I knew that was difficult for some. You had never to forget that you had come to see Limey and to give him full attention. I have seen friends and relatives gathered together in a sickroom, totally ignoring the patient, talking among themselves as if the person in the bed didn't exist, sometimes as if he couldn't hear or was already dead. We talked to Limey, and about his interests. We did not ignore his physical handicaps, but we also talked about his poetry, about food and gardens, about politics and books.

I had brought to his room a copy of the book he had edited, abridged, and translated from the French, Alexandre Dumas' *Dictionary of Cuisine* (Simon and Schuster, 1958). As the dust jacket explained, "The great fortune Dumas made from writing his five hundred books was spent on women and food. . . . The *Grand Dictionnaire de Cuisine* on which Dumas worked in the final years of his life was first published posthumously in 1873. The original uncut French book has been almost unobtainable for many years." Limey had discovered the book in French, and had had a marvelous time working on it. He still enjoyed hearing some of the wild recipes, such as the one for "Poached Eggs" (fifteen of them), which required roasting twelve ducks on a spit, cutting them to the bone, and draining off their juices. The juice was then seasoned with salt and coarse pepper, reheated, but not boiled, and poured over the eggs. This recipe was followed by one entitled "Poached Eggs without Duck Juice."

I had also brought up a copy of a book we had had a good time working on together, *The Country Week End Cookbook* (M. Barrows & Co., 1961). Limey particularly wanted this to show to the dietitian, in the hope, I suppose, that she might find in it some more interesting menus than what he had been getting. We used to get up early in the morning when we were writing that book and start right in. By around ten o'clock, in spite of an ample breakfast, we were so starving from talking about food that I'd have to stop and make hamburgers for us both. As a matter of fact, I suspect we ate up the profits of that book before it was even finished.

Limey also began to talk about writing a book, a sequel to his one novel, *Lumber*. For me this was so remarkable and sad that I didn't know how to handle it. We had always talked about our writing—Limey had always read my manuscripts before I sent them out and had given me his voluminous notes to read, as he had written them, during the five years after his first stroke. Now there was a time lapse between his dictating into the tape recorder and my finding someone to do the transcribing. I was relieved, a couple of weeks after he first spoke about the book, to see that he had dictated a letter to two writer friends, thereby relieving me of the burden of having to discuss such a heartbreaking and impossible fantasy with him.

He wrote:

Dear Ring or Ian or both,
I think attached to this are some pages of transcript dealing with a novel to be called "What Happened to Pearl." I must say at this point that after the publication of my novel "Lumber" in 1931, Little, Brown and Company, at the end of which the bloody remains of Jimmy Logan (the protagonist of "Lumber") were dumped on the porch in front of his wife Pearl, and she cracked up—after that I got very concerned about Pearl as though she were a completely independent person without anything to do with the story "Lumber" at all, and I used to worry about her and wonder what the hell happened to her.

Now I think I want to write the story of what happened to Pearl and I have made some notes on it somewhere in the enclosed transcriptions and one piece of paper that I typed myself. But I find myself unable to organize the damned thing, chiefly because I can't read notes. My vision doesn't encompass the normal eight and a half inches of a typewritten line, and so I am asking you to do what you would with it, if you want to. I place no restrictions on what you do with it; you can throw it away if you want. You can even use it for movie material if that's what you wish, although in general I have no desire for any movie credits at all. Or, of course, an obvious treatment for this would be to quote the last few paragraphs of "Lumber" and then go ahead with the synopsis of the story. In any case, I can't do this myself and I'm asking you guys to help me out somehow or other with this goddam thing. I need a lot of help and I trust to the goodness of your hearts to do the best you can with it, whatever that may be and whatever form it may take. And I love you and trust you.

Of course, nothing ever happened, and Limey himself, once he had dictated the letter and a few notes, seemed to drop it. I was rather frightened and upset by the whole incident because, while the fact that he was even thinking about writing a book was in itself incredible, it gave me a glimpse of the world of fantasy in which he was living. Did he really believe that he was going to write a book? I am inclined to think, his confusion lay in not remembering what he had actually dictated and what he had only thought out in his mind but never got to put on the tapes. Because of a few things that he said later, I don't think that he actually forgot about Pearl Logan, but that he was writing her story in his mind many times while he was lying in bed, and perhaps that was enough to satisfy him.

We did a lot of reminiscing. Limey's mind had turned to his past a great deal, back to his early childhood, to his parents, to his youthful years in lumber mills, to crossing the country on freight cars, to his first wife, who had died when they were both in their twenties.

I was not always happy with his reminiscing. I had a terrible dread of its being a sign of senility, the way very old people seem to live in the past. It was, I suppose, a partly justified dread, and yet my wanting him to live in the present was ridiculous. His present was obviously agonizing and he certainly had nothing to look for in the future. Limey's dwelling so much in his past was depressing for me. I wanted to hold on to Limey, and when he slipped back into that world before I knew him, I felt that I was losing him. He romanticized his past. Even his father, whom he had always painted as a fanatic and a tyrant—a man who one Sunday Christmas morning, when Limey was ten or eleven years old, had taken him down to the cellar and thrown a Christmas gift book into the furnace because Limey had dared to read it on the Sabbath, when only the Bible was allowed. The worst thing I had ever done to Limey in the years of our marriage was once, in a fit of anger, to yell at him, "You sound just like your father." I'm not sure he ever forgave me for that, and now I was illogically furious that he was forgiving the man whose iron hand, in so many ways, had been laid on him even from the grave.

Or perhaps it wasn't that I was angry with Limey for

forgiving his father, but that I was angry at having to deal with emotions of my own that were irrelevant to his getting better. I was jealous of Limey's past, although God knows I had had one of my own. But Limey had been forty when I met him, and now, suddenly, I was angry that I had missed all those good years when he had been active and healthy, his bohemian years of wandering, and those few years his first love, his first wife, had shared with him. Suddenly our thirty years together seemed so short. I was on a single track; I didn't want my mixed and often confused feelings about Limey's past brought out at that time, and I resented it when they were. It was a foolish resentment. Limey's preoccupation with his past was as much a symptom of his illness as his inability to move his body; if you can patiently feed a man in his seventies, you must also develop the patience to listen to what he wants to say, and you cannot always choose the subject.

Patience, patience . . . that was never my forte. In all my life I'd always done everything in a hurry. I knew Limey three weeks before I married him; we looked at our house about ten minutes before we put a deposit on it. I walk fast, I write fast, and I hate waiting. But with a stroke patient, it's waiting, and waiting some more. It seems to me that those days I was waiting more than ever before. Every time the phone rang I jumped for fear it was the nursing home calling to tell me that something had happened to Limey. Never anything good. But what? Was I expecting him to die? Was some part of my unconscious hoping for it? I don't know, but I don't really think so. I wanted very much to have him home. But not until the professionals had taught him to handle himself better.

Like any institution, a nursing home is as good as its staff. We have a weakness in this country for impressive physical plants: multimillion-dollar schools with great lawns and shade trees; sprawling modern factories that boards of trustees can show off. We are always building monuments of brick and mortar. I'd like to see more money spent on what goes on inside. I've seen beautiful, airy libraries in schools where the shelves were empty because there was no money left in the budget for books. And the men and women who work in nursing homes are probably among the most underpaid people you can find anywhere. The work is hard, it can be very unpleasant, and I sometimes wonder why anyone wants to do it. I admire them all.

But the plight of the staff was not my problem at that moment, and I was pretty disturbed to see their interest in Limey running out. I use the word "interest" because I think that is exactly what happened. In the beginning Limey was someone new, the nurses and aides found him interesting and amusing, but the tediousness of taking care of him won out. He was not easy to take care of. He had to be fed, he had to be cleaned, he had to be dressed and undressed, he had to be washed and shaved, he had to be lifted into the wheelchair, wheeled, and then lifted back into bed. They gave him a urinal, but his bed had to be changed often when he didn't get it in time. When he was in bed he was supposed to be turned every couple of hours from one side to the other. And at regular intervals he had to be given medication.

Limey was also a great disappointment, I think, because he was not improving. For those whose work is dedicated to making people well, a patient who fails to respond to treatment presents the doctor with a discouraging and frustrating reminder of his own fallibility. Doctors like to make people well, and properly take pride when they succeed in doing so. But no one was able to give Limey good marks for improvement. Like poor learners in school, the aging and the chronically ill are not a source of gratification for those professionals who care for them, and I believe the patients suffer because of it. I do not know what the answer is, since doctors as well as teachers are humans first, but I felt the syndrome creeping in. I was not writing Limey off, and the discouragement I saw in the faces of the staff frightened me.

And so I was disturbed but not too surprised when I found that there were days when they did not get him out of bed, although the doctors had stressed the importance of that. If he was not moved regularly, his limbs could become totally stiff, so that his knees would not bend at all and he could not be put into a sitting position. He might become like a wooden board. When he had howled about staying in the wheelchair, he had been told, "If we let you stay in bed you won't be able to move. You'll be a million times worse." There were also days now when they did not get him dressed, and while often his mood was better when he was in bed, I was discouraged.

I did get upset, however, when after a few weeks I saw that nothing had been done about training him to be pivoted from the bed to the wheelchair. I had been told that this could be done by even a small, slight person, once you knew how. I was annoyed that little progress had been made in teaching him to feed himself. I had brought him a box of cherries, a fruit he liked enormously, and had spent an afternoon insisting that he pick up each cherry himself and put it in his mouth. It was a painstaking, shattering process to watch, but he did it, and while he said, "It's easier if you feed me," I'm sure he did get satisfaction out of it. I'd felt as excited then as when I'd sold my first story.

I asked for a conference with the physical therapist and the occupational therapist. I have to admit that I had some paranoia about being aggressive, with all the pejorative connotations that term has come to hold. But I didn't care—dammit, I was fighting for my husband's life and my own. The paranoia came from the cloud under which Medicare is shrouded. Medicare comes under the Social Security Act and is not charity; nor, I might add, is Medicaid. Medicaid is a federal program for persons whose income puts them in the poverty class (as set by the government) and covers various illnesses and handicaps regardless of age. Medicaid has to be applied for and eligibility has varied from year to year, with the trend being to cut down services rather than expand. To my mind, it is no more a charity than having a fire truck and firemen come to put a fire out when your house is burning. My uneducated guess is that more than 90 percent of the patients in nursing homes are paid for by either Medicare or Medicaid.

But this country is so gung-ho on private enterprise, and has been told so often that government programs are handouts, that many of us who have been used to paying our own way have become victims of a terrible brain-washing: if we're not paying for something directly out of our own pockets, we are supposed to accept meekly what is offered. My response to that, bluntly, was bullshit.

My reasoning, however, did not prevent me from feeling childishly apologetic when talking with the two amiable young women therapists, having to add to my qualms about being a recipient of charity the intimidation of the layman speaking to professionals. They told me their problems, I told them mine, and yes, they did understand and would certainly do something about it.

It soon turned out that if anything was going to be done, it would have to be done promptly. I came in one day when Limey had been there for about three or four weeks and found a message asking me to see the social worker. My heart fell. Social workers did not spell good news for me. I was directed to an office where once again I sat across the desk from a young woman. (They all seemed to be young!) "Your husband's Medicare payments are running out," she told me. "We're having a hard time now justifying his staying here." I had to listen politely to a familiar story. Medicare, Part B, pays for only a limited stay in a nursing home, the average being around four or five weeks. They will not pay for custodial care, etc., etc. "Your husband is a very sick man," she ended up. "I'm not saying he has to go home tomorrow, but it probably will be in another week or so. What are your plans for him?"

My plans for him . . . my plans are to wave a magic wand to make him well, to go back to Florida, and never to see a social worker or a nursing home again for the rest of my life. My plans are to slit my throat. My plans are to weep for all the helpless people in the world, and their sisters and their cousins and their aunts.

"To take him home," I said brightly. "What are my choices?"

"I don't think you can take care of him at home. He needs a great deal of care."

"What do you suggest?"

The amiable young woman fidgeted in her seat. She was a well-groomed, carefully coiffed woman who lived in a home, I was sure, that was shining bright. "Have you thought about keeping him in a nursing home?"

"How much is it a day here?"

She came up with a figure that I quickly multiplied in my head by 360, and arrived at an annual cost, not including therapy, medication, or doctors, that would consume almost all of our income, provided I was able to continue to write as much as I had been doing.

"I've thought about it a lot," I said, "but I'm afraid we don't have that kind of money. Besides, I think he'd be happier at home."

"You have to think about yourself. You're a young, active woman, you have to live too. You know"—she looked at me thoughtfully, and, once more, I knew what was coming—"you could put whatever assets you have in your name and divorce him. Then he could go on Medicaid. It would only be a technicality . . ."

I looked that woman straight in the eye and I thought, "I'm going to say it this time, I'm really going to say it," but I didn't. I did stare at the wedding ring on her finger, however, and I thought, "I'll bet you didn't let your husband come near you before that little technicality of a wedding ceremony was performed, and if you ever have a daughter you'd be the one to scream the loudest if she should live with a man without benefit of clergy. How dare you sit there and tell me to divorce my husband when I love him, when he's sick, maybe dying . . . sit there and tell me in your cool voice that my marriage is a technicality that I can undo to suit insane, idiotic laws? How dare you?"

Why waste my breath? I got out of that room as fast as I could, got into my car, and started driving. I drove furiously for about half an hour and then I pulled over to the side of the road and I wept. I cried as I hadn't for days. I really sobbed, with my whole body shaking, cries of anger, of frustration, of sorrow.

If there is such a thing as a "good cry," maybe that was it, for it set me off on a lot of hard thinking. You can get so caught up and involved with the daily problems—waking up every morning to the same pain, wondering how is Limey, what is truly going through his mind, how are you going to work and go to the nursing home, wandering aimlessly around the house alone, packing a bag of clean clothes for him, answering the telephone, paying bills, using up so much emotional energy every day that you lose sight of the whole picture. But now the thought that had been lurking about in my subconscious suddenly surfaced, full-blown: that nursing home was not really the best place for Limey. The beautiful surroundings that it offered he could not make use of (he never once got into that cheerful dining room), and the physical therapy, done on the bed (there was no gym as in the hospital), did not seem more than we could do at home. Superior as this convalescent home was, and I believe it is as fine a one as can be found anywhere, it was still an institution that had a negative psychological effect on both Limey and me. So now, anxious as I had been to get him in, I was as eager to get him out and home.

But I had a lot of things to do before that would be possible. My first step was to call our family doctor and tell him that Limey was coming home, that I wanted Limey to be under his care, and that I needed his advice on where to get help. He told me to call the Visiting Nurse Association. I will say right here that this was one of the most useful calls I ever made. The VNA in our area serviced several towns, and I was put on to the nurse who took care of ours. She told me that the nursing home would send a medical report to our doctor and would also fill out forms for the VNA and send them to their office. When my husband came home the VNA would work directly under the supervision of our local doctor. The best news was that the nurse would visit Limey at least once a week, that a physical therapist would also come to the house once a week (we were to do the daily exercises she would show us), and that the office hoped to get me a nurse's aide, if one was available, to come four hours a day, five days a week. We discussed the equipment we would need, but they did not have much, although she thought our town owned a hospital bed that I should find out about. The nursing care and the therapist would be covered by Medicare as long as Limey needed them. I did not feel so alone, and I had my fingers crossed about the nurse's aide.

Next I went to see our First Selectman, a genial, considerate man. Yes, he said, there was a hospital bed somewhere in town and he'd find out where it was. He wasn't sure there was an over-the-bed table. I was beginning to discover that if you are in trouble, there is nothing like a small town, and certainly none like ours. Everyone wanted to help. I cannot overemphasize the comfort I got from the practical assistance that was given me. I was not shy about asking around for what I needed because everyone was so straightforward about wanting to give. I found, though, that it was a help to know what I needed and to be specific in my requests.

Alone in the house, I studied where to put Limey. I was getting very excited about his homecoming and I wanted everything to be ready and right. I didn't have much choice about rooms: there was either his study, where all his books and his desk and manuscripts were, or our guest room. I opted for the guest room. It was larger and had a lot of windows. Actually I had been avoiding Limey's study, so full of his work, and if I found it depressing, it could be much worse for him.

Each time we had added on to our house, it seemed the
new floor had to be on a different level, so that various
sets of two and three steps were scattered about our one-
story house. That meant that if I didn't want Limey con-
fined to the bedroom, I would have to get ramps built for
his wheelchair. I hired a carpenter and together we also
worked out a removable ramp for our front door so that
we could take him outside on our terrace.

Much to my surprise, within a few days everything was
falling into place. Good friends in New York said they
had what they called the Cadillac of wheelchairs and
would bring it up to the country for Limey. The VNA had
a nurse's aide lined up to come in from noon until four,
five days a week. The foreman of the town crew called to
say they had the hospital bed and would bring it over
whenever I said. I rented an over-the-bed table for a
month—if it proved useful (which it did), I could then
buy it.

My friend Lois came over with an armful of gifts. We
laughed about the assortment: not flowers or books or
caviar and champagne. She brought a bedpan, a urinal,
some elegant sheets, and a huge roll of Chucks (absor-
bent, disposable bed pads used in hospitals), which I had
discovered cost a fortune at the pharmacy, if they could
get them for me. She also told me to buy some flannelette
crib sheets and boxes of Pampers. We did not intend to
wrap Limey up in diapers but to use the disposable
Pampers as top padding under his rear end. I added to the
collection a large can of baby powder and some Vaseline
Intensive Care Lotion. The curtains were washed, the

furniture in the room disposed of, and the hospital bed brought in.

One very important item on my list, however, still had to be taken care of: to find someone to come in during the mornings and for some part of the weekends. Eager as I was for Limey to come home, I was also nervous. I had been nervous when I had first brought my tiny babies home from the hospital, and this was much worse. Although Limey had lost a lot of weight, he was a tall man, his body was dead weight, and I could not possibly move him alone. That last week in the nursing home they had started to pivot him from the bed to the wheelchair, and back again, but I saw that even with those experienced people it took two to move him. The procedure was for Limey to be swung around to the edge of the bed, sitting up with his feet firmly on the floor, with a person sitting on either side of him for support. The wheelchair, with the brake on, was set at right angles to the bed, and then those holding him would gently swing him around from sitting on the bed to sitting in the wheelchair. It was a tricky procedure, and there was always the danger that he would land on the floor. I had been brainwashed by the doctors to be quite fanatical about getting him out of bed every day, and—since he could not tolerate the wheelchair for too long—twice a day if possible.

I did not need a nurse, but rather a strong, willing, and kind person, male or female. I don't remember how many telephone calls I made, following up one lead after another. My thought was to find someone on social security who wanted to work part-time for the extra money.

As I might have known, the person I finally found was one whose name had been given me by the people in our one store, the center of all information in town. She turned out to be a tall, imposing-looking middle-aged woman who lived not far from us, who had had some experience taking care of sick people, and who appeared anxious for the job. We agreed on an hourly salary and for her to come in five mornings from eight until noon; we would work out the weekends depending on whether our sons and their families would be around or not.

When the word came that Medicare for the nursing home was to be cut off, I was not sorry. My euphoria about bringing Limey home was hard to explain to anyone. Even our sons asked a few times, "Mother, are you sure you know what you are doing?" Our neurologist, Dr. Wolf, was skeptical. Our friends, I believe, thought I was quite mad. One dear friend went so far as to sit down with me to discuss finances. We figured out how much help at home would cost for a year, and then she made out a list of people to whom she would go to ask for contributions to pay the difference between that and the cost of a nursing home. I told her to put the list away, just in case, for some future date. One of the warmest things that happened was a note I got from a close friend in town with a list of the names and telephone numbers of approximately fifteen people—all of whom she had contacted—who wanted to be called to come and sit with Limey in the evening so that I could get out to a movie or a dinner or whatever. I broke up when I read that.

The morning the ambulance was to come to pick me

up to go and get Limey I was up early. I washed my hair, I put flowers around, I even brushed Jo, the crazy poodle, and I laid fires in both fireplaces. I was as nervous and excited as a bride. What Limey had talked about for these past months was going to happen: we were going to sit by our own fireside and have a drink together. So what if he would be sitting in a wheelchair; he'd be here in our own house, which he loved so much, and not in a dismal hospital or a distant nursing home.

The ambulance came on schedule, and we set out. It is amazing to me, the tricks the mind (or the emotions?) play. Each time I went to see Limey I was shocked anew by his condition. This time was no exception. There was no logical reason for me to expect anything different, yet I did. I had not given it any special thought, but I just naturally expected a response to my enthusiasm, to the fact that he was coming home. Limey was not bubbly. He was, if anything, more despondent than usual.

"Why don't you let me stay here?" was his greeting.

"Don't you want to come home? I thought you'd be so happy."

"Yes, I'd like to be home, but . . ." His eyes averted mine. "You won't be able to take care of me."

"We'll have the nurse's aide, and I have a very good woman hired. It's going to work fine."

"It's going to be too much of a burden for you."

"Don't say that, please. I want you home. It's been so lonesome without you."

"Why don't you let me die?"

"You're not dying." I spoke fiercely. I couldn't bear that conversation. I couldn't stand the cold water he was dumping on me, and I hated feeling so let down. As so often, I had been so involved with my own feelings and let myself get so excited that I had not given a thought to his feelings. Limey was terrified of coming home.

Believe me, I did not realize that instantly. It took several dreadful days, I think the worst days of his entire illness. After all, he had been treating the nursing home as someplace temporary, and had talked so wistfully about wanting to be home. That he would be afraid to come home had never occurred to me. I can see now that it must have loomed before him as a gigantic step, which indeed it was. On the objective side, he was leaving the safety and security of the care of professional people, registered nurses within call, a doctor on call, aides to administer to him, emergency equipment on hand. All the small things that were taken care of automatically by the nursing staff and that he obviously feared no one would be able to do for him at home: changing his bed sheets as often as necessary, often several times a day; giving him his therapy; feeding him; changing his position; washing and shaving him; keeping his body clear of bed sores; and taking care of his incontinence. In the latter department, Limey was quite extraordinary. He was a very private person, yet he accepted natural functions of the body as a matter of course. He hated having his backside cleaned, and he loathed a bedpan, but he was much less bothered by his incontinence than I would have expected him to be. "I think there's a lot of shit there," he would say when he wanted to be cleaned, and because of his paralysis, he often did not know whether there was or there wasn't. But he made no fuss about the indignity of it, accepting the fact of life that if one ate, one defecated.

On the subjective side, he was terribly concerned about being a burden to me. He was the kind of man who, whenever he had been sick, wanted to crawl into a hole and be left alone. He had never wanted to be waited on, sick or well. He had always put great stock in his self-sufficiency, secure in the knowledge that he could market, cook for himself, take care of a house—no woman had to "do" for him. (Which, of course, had suited me very well.) But now, being put into the position of having to be taken care of by me, his wife, a woman who in the past had rejected the notion of slavishly catering to a man, must have been abhorrent to him. And I think he was truly worried that he could not be properly taken care of at home. Then there was his own dream of walking back into our house, not of being carried in on a stretcher. As a matter of fact, he had said a few times, "I walked into that hospital when I came up from Florida, I'm going to get out of bed and walk now. You're just keeping me in bed. Where's my cane? Give me my cane."

But that was the least of what he said. Limey came home on a Friday, and in my euphoria I had deliberately not asked any help to come in that day. I had imagined a lovely day at home, alone, with Limey. Our younger son was coming on Saturday for the weekend, and I figured that between the two of us we could do what was needed, and that Monday would be time enough to break in new people and start our routine.

I don't know, and never will, whether Limey was honestly confused because of the change from one place to another, or whether he was testing me, but I can mark that weekend down as the worst I have ever spent in my life. He didn't let up for a minute with either Jimmy or me, and especially me.

I had not been prepared for his hostility, for his fury at his own helplessness, for his tremendous anger, for his fears, or for the fact that, obviously, I had to be the butt of all his feelings. If I'd had a brain in my head I should have known, instead of being swept up in all my la-de-da goings-on with fresh flowers, and expensive fresh salmon for his supper, and a nostalgic dream of a fireside chat. I imagine that the reality was worse just because I had let myself be so carried away, and my only excuse for my awful behavior was that I was totally unprepared.

We fought the whole weekend. And I mean fought. At one point I came so close to giving him a slap on his behind that I was terrified of my own reaction. One minute he would say, "Why don't you let me die?" and then, if I left him alone in his room for a few minutes, he'd ring the bell we had hitched up for him and bring me on the run. "You're abandoning me, you're leaving me."

The bell rang incessantly. Very often because he felt like ringing it. "But, Limey, if you keep ringing the bell I won't know when you really need me."

"I know," he said, and kept on ringing.

"Tell Jimmy I want to see him," he said.

"Jimmy's coming tomorrow."

A few minutes later: "Morris is outside. Tell him to come in."

"Morris isn't here."

"He is here. I know he's here. I want to see him."

He kept trapping me into arguments. He would ask for the urinal, and I'd give it to him. A few minutes later he would ask for it again, and I'd tell him he had just used it. He'd insist he hadn't, and I'd give it to him again. Then he'd complain that I never took it away. He didn't like the salmon (usually a great favorite of his) and complained it was too dry, although it was in a dill and sour cream sauce. He wanted his pillow moved, he tried getting out of bed and only succeeded in kicking his covers off with his right leg, getting it over the side of the bed and scaring me sick. He howled, really howled, when I had to clean him. He was furiously angry, like a small child, when I had to answer the phone. When I put my arms around him he said that I was hurting him. He rejected me in every way he could.

The night was a nightmare. He stayed awake, in spite of Valium (I had been told not to give him a sleeping pill), and kept me awake the entire night, calling me, complaining, saying that he wanted to die, accusing me of abandoning him . . . there was no letup. When Jimmy arrived on Saturday there was no improvement. He let us get him into the wheelchair, screaming all the while. "You're both so rough, you don't know how to do it," despite the fact that we had thought we'd managed a smooth, gentle transfer. We wheeled him out to the porch, but he was there only five minutes when he started to bang on the chair with the one arm he could move, and howled. I cannot describe that howl of his. It sounded more animal than human, and it tore at my heart. I begged him, sobbing, to please stop. I couldn't bear it. Jimmy yelled at him to behave himself. We both yelled at him that day and that night, when he kept us both up again.

When Jimmy had to leave on Sunday we were both in despair. "You can't do it, Mom," Jimmy said. On the phone Jonny told me the same thing. I was ready to agree with them, but what choice did I have? "I've got to give it a try," I told them, told myself.

On Monday morning Mrs. Thorpe arrived, looking more professional in her starched white dress than she turned out to be. I spent the morning with her, showing her what had to be done: preparing his breakfast, bathing him, dressing him, and, with my help, getting him into the wheelchair, then, after lunch when the nurse's aide arrived, getting him back to bed. It sounds easy on paper. Limey had brought home with him from the nursing home a special spoon that would supposedly enable him to feed himself. But it was poorly designed: it was too deep, and while it was made to slide a little on the handle, it slid so that the food fell off before he got it to his mouth. I dug up a more shallow sugar spoon, which he was able to manage with some degree of success, although plenty of food dropped on to the bib we tied on him. We also tried to give him food, such as cheese and cut-up meat, that he could pick up and eat with his fingers if he worked at it. Watching Limey feed himself was a trial of patience, and one of the hardest things was to get the people who took care of him to do it. It was much easier to feed him. I had to keep after them constantly because the therapist said it was important, and it seemed so to me. Limey himself was ambivalent. One part of him, I believe, wanted to do as much as he could himself; whatever he did, however, took an enormous effort, so there could be no hard-and-fast rule. Often he asked to be fed. Good judgment had to be used, and that was hard to come by. This meant that I felt impelled to be around for as many of his meals as possible.

The nurse's aide turned out to be a darling, and Limey immediately responded to her professionalism. It was after she was there and I saw Limey's reaction that it began to dawn on me that he honestly had been afraid that I was going to take care of him myself, that I would not be able to, that I would not like it, and that the burden of having him home was going to be too much and I would eventually resent it. I might have avoided that weekend if I had had help right away. It never occurred to me that Limey could not assimilate what I told him was going to happen in a few days—that it was only the right now that he understood. I said earlier that I believed a spouse is better off working than acting as nurse, and I now realized that it was important from the patient's point of view as well. It is much easier for a patient to deal with a stranger, with someone who is paid for a job, than to have all the emotional problems connected with a dependency on someone close. I think I could have saved myself considerable grief if I hadn't romanticized Limey's condition, and also, I confess, fantasized the role of Omniscient Wife. I was going to welcome him home, and show him how much I loved him by doing it all myself the first few days.

That the homecoming was such a fiasco was also a result of the fact that, since Limey was central to me, I wanted to be central to him, but I had picked out a mechanical way to do it. Since Limey had always been capable around the house, and had never wanted to be waited upon by me, I don't know why I thought he would want it now. There were other things he wanted from me, which were more important, and that I was better equipped to give. It didn't take me long to learn what they were, but immediate, practical problems had to be solved first.

On Tuesday I was ready to settle into a routine: to get Mrs. Thorpe started at eight in the morning and then to get to work at my typewriter. When she was ready to get Limey into the wheelchair I would come out of the study to help her and show her what to fix for his lunch. My plan was that from noon until four, when the nurse's aide had to leave, I would have some free time. I could do my shopping, go to the library, go for a walk, have lunch with a friend, or work some more if I wanted to. Since Limey usually slept after his lunch, we decided not to get him up again in the afternoon on a regular basis—if guests were coming to see him, the nurse's aide and I would get him up and the visitor, if it was someone I could ask to do this, would help me get him back to bed.

(Some friends, I knew, would be too upset or nervous.) After four I was on my own.

It was a fine plan, and it actually worked part of the time. That Tuesday the morning was shot. Our family doctor came out to check Limey over—he had not seen him since his massive stroke. The visiting nurse and the physical therapist also came. Limey's greeting to our doctor was "Bill, give me the needle. I'm ready for it."

Bill gave his rueful smile. "Sorry, I can't do it. I'd go to jail and I don't think I want to do that." Bill gave him no Pollyanna talk, and that was the basis of Limey's affection for him. Bill had no new information to add about his medical condition and, like the other doctors, he said that the nurses knew more about taking care of his bowels than he did. The therapist showed Mrs. Thorpe and me the exercises to give Limey every morning and every night, and said she would come back again to show them to the nurse's aide.

The visiting nurse and the therapist were warm, intelligent, fine women who gave me as much moral support as practical help. I think they truly liked Limey and were sincerely concerned about how I was holding up. They succeeded in making me feel that I was doing pretty well. We laughed and chatted together with the quick intimacy of persons aware of a grim situation, doing what had to be done but refusing to let it take over. I remember once trying to get a urinal to stay in place when someone said, "I hope you're enjoying all these women fooling around with your penis." Limey's reply was "I never liked group sex. I prefer one woman at a time." Limey's attitude about sex, as it was about his incontinence, was as free from inhibitions or false modesty as it ever had been. He would sometimes glance at his limp penis and say, "Poor thing, I guess it's had its day. But they were good days, or nights, I should say. It had its fun."

That afternoon when everyone had left, I felt truly close to Limey for the first time since he had gotten ill. I stretched out on the bed beside him, and we lay quietly, looking out to our woods, and to Jo running around in her roomy runway. Our bodies were side by side, his under the covers, mine not, and it was as if the sexuality between us had entered a new phase. There would never again be a sexual act between his wounded body and mine, and yet there was a peacefulness in our closeness that seemed to me a poignant aftermath, a gentle release from the turbulent sex we had enjoyed over the years. I felt that nature had handed me an unexpected bonus in allowing me to feel so at rest just lying beside Limey. I think he felt it too, for he wanted me to stay close, and after a while he spoke quietly about us, about our children, about our life together, the way people sometimes do after making love. It was a small time like this, about which I could not tell anyone, that assured me that, despite all the problems of having him at home, it was the only way.

Later, when I talked with our sons about Limey and his illness, they told me that I seemed able to get some gratification they could not. And they were right. Because they came on visits, were not living with him, they could not get past the physical aspects. It took more than even a weekend, and of course their relationship with Limey was different from mine. But the warm, familiar times I had with Limey alone more than made up for the difficulties and made having him home totally worthwhile.

I had bought a small television set and put it on the wall where he could see it. At six o'clock we watched the news together while I had a drink. I enjoyed giving him his supper, washing him, and getting him ready for the night. I went to bed that night feeling better than I had in months.

I still felt good the next morning, and eager to get to work. I turned on the "Today" show for Limey, a show he asked for every morning, and went about my business of showering and breakfast. Since Limey was occupied watching the box, I decided to leave his care to Mrs. Thorpe when she arrived at eight. Eight o'clock, no Mrs. Thorpe. Eight-fifteen, no sign of her. By eight-thirty I called her up. "Oh, I'm not coming in. I can't do all that bending. My back hurts."

"Why didn't you call me?" I demanded.

"I was going to later," she said casually.

"Does this mean you're not coming back?"

"I told you, it hurts my back. I'll come by and pick up the two days you owe me."

"Thanks a lot." I banged down the phone. And I panicked. I remembered saying to a friend, "When you have a big problem, the small ones aren't that important anymore. They fall into place." Was I ever eating those words! I felt furious, helpless, and close to calling up our

sons and saying, "I can't cope. I'm going to have a nervous breakdown and you will have to take over. You
make the decisions, he's your father, you take care of him,
I can't do it."

I didn't do that. A spouse is responsible for a spouse
. . . children have their own lives to lead . . . all the
good old clichés came to mind with little comfort. I was
back at the beginning, loathing a society in which I could
not have a trained, professional, reliable, full-time person
for home nursing care, a service that would be cheaper
and better than keeping him in an institution which was
now available only to the very rich and the indigent.
What insanity.

I took care of Limey that morning, and in order not to
vent my anger on him, poor darling, I picked on the first
name that came to mind: Happy Rockefeller. I guess the
name Rockefeller was enough. She would never know
that for one morning she was the butt of a distraught
woman's frustration at the unfairness of a free society in
which some people are more free than others.

Cynical Limey was amused by my mutterings. "There
was a time when anyone with the name Rockefeller
couldn't be elected to dog catcher in this country, but
what did Happy do to you?" Limey thought it pretty
funny that *mit en drenen* (in the middle of everything),
as he said, I should be mad at Happy Rockefeller.

"Nothing. Never laid eyes on the woman. But she can
hire nurses by the carload, and I bet I'm smarter than she
is. I've written a lot of good books, but am I rich? No." I

was mad enough not to want to make sense and by the time the nurse's aide arrived at noon I was laughing at my one-sided battle.

But what was I going to do? I got busy on the phone again, went up to the store, got some more names to call, and switched my frustration from people to a mechanical object that gave me a busy signal, or no answer, or a negative response. It wasn't fun and it wasn't funny. I would be totally licked if I couldn't find help. I had to be able to work, but it was more than that.

Limey had never been an easy man, and he was not an easy patient. A stroke, and I suppose any long illness, does change one's personality. From a rather quiet person Limey was turning into a compulsive talker. His chattering could be unnerving because he went through certain patterns and routines repeatedly. He was aware of it, and often said, "I'm talking too much, aren't I?"

"Sometimes you are," I told him, but apparently he couldn't stop himself. My feelings, as they were about so many things, were mixed. Hearing him talk so much was reassuring in one way, but it could also drive me nuts.

He had a habit of verbalizing everything we did for him; although we did the same thing every day and knew what we were doing, he had to tell us each move. When we were getting him dressed: "Now put on my shirt."

"Yes. I'm putting on your shirt."

"You can't do it. You won't get my arm through the sleeve."

"It will come through. Just take it easy. We get it on every day."

"Don't forget to put on my socks."

"No, we won't forget."

That conversation went on all through the dressing. Then, when we wanted to get him into the wheelchair: "You have to put the wheelchair over here, next to the bed."

"Yes, I know."

"Put on the brake."

"It's on. Come now, we're going to swing you around."

"I can't. I can't do it. I'll fall."

"No, you won't fall. We have hold of you. Put your feet on the floor."

"They're on the floor."

"No, they're not. Put them down, keep your right foot down." He was swinging his right foot. "You have to keep it down."

"Hila, sit down beside me."

"Yes, of course, I'm sitting beside you."

"You won't be able to put me on the chair. You'll bump me."

"We'll do our best. Are you ready now? Keep your feet on the floor."

"I'm slipping, I'm falling . . ."

"No, you're not. You're sitting up fine. Try and relax. We'll sit here for a minute or two before we move you."

"I can't relax. I never relax. Sit close to me, Hila."

"I'm very close. I have my arm around you . . ." I kissed his cheek. "Now, one, two, three, let's go . . ."

We swung him around neatly into the chair. But no matter how smoothly it went, it was never smooth enough for him. "That was a hard bump. Only Charlie does it right." Charlie was my neighbor's caretaker, who was a dear man and often came to help if I or the nurse's aide, or someone working for me, was alone. Once in the chair, Limey had to tell us how to put his legs up, how to attach the tray a friend had made to rest his arms on, how to turn his chair around.

Remember that we went through the process of moving Limey at least twice every day, from bed to wheelchair and back again, and very often four times, when we got him up in the afternoon as well as the morning. Then he directed us all the way in getting the chair down the ramp and through our narrow hall (never made for a wheelchair) and into a front room. "Don't go fast . . . you'll never get through the door . . . tell me when there's a bump . . . you're shaking me too much . . ." No matter how many hundreds of times we did it we heard the same patter.

No sooner had I settled him near a window, but not near enough for the light to hurt his eyes, given him his tape recorder, and gone in to try to work, than he started calling for his lunch. "You just had your breakfast. It's not even ten o'clock. I'll give you some juice, but not lunch yet."

I knew why he wanted his lunch. After lunch he could go back to bed, and that's what he wanted. Any excuse to get out of the wheelchair.

Someone asked, "Has Limey's sense of time been affected?" It is hard to say whether his sense of time was affected by the stroke or simply by the fact of having been in bed for so long a time. Early on, when he was first in the hospital, one of the doctors said, "When I'm in bed for a week I lose all sense of time—that can happen to anyone." I have also been asked, "What exactly does happen when you have a stroke?" That is an impossible question, as no two stroke patients are exactly alike. Every single thought or movement a person makes, from the flick of an eye to throwing a ball, from uttering a sound to working out a mathematical problem, is directed by the brain. And since these directions come from thousands of different cells in the brain, the particular cells or combination of cells that are affected by a stroke (the loss of blood flowing to those cells) will determine the patient's impairments, and these will obviously vary from person to person.

By recording the difficulties involved in taking care of Limey I am not trying to prove that I was a saint, but precisely the opposite. I had to recognize my own limitations, and I knew that I could not cope with his daily routine. To learn in a situation like mine what you can do and what you cannot is a process of trial and error, and you are wise to find out. Obviously I could not eliminate all that was unpleasant or difficult—for instance, unless I made special arrangements, I had always to be on hand to help anyone working for me to move Limey. But for his sake and mine I was not going to settle for having someone in the house only four hours a day. I loved that man, and it was painful to hear him chatter on (something he had always loathed in other people), and the temptation to yell at him to shut up could become obsessive.

As I write about the difficulties, I remember also how much of his good nature, his generosity and tenderness, Limey retained. He had always had very sharp ears, and his hearing had not been impaired at all. There were times when he overheard me on the phone (two rooms removed) telling someone that I did not want to go out because I didn't want to leave him alone. No sooner did I hang up than he called me. "Don't stay home because of me. Go out, you need it. I'll be okay, I don't mind being alone. Go out and have a good time, have a martini for me." Very occasionally, when I was going someplace close by, I would leave him for an hour or two, but I never felt comfortable, and I did it very rarely, although short of a fire nothing could happen to him when he was in bed.

Limey had loved buying presents. As much as he hated shopping, he always came with me to shop for Christmas presents for our kids and grandchildren and took great pleasure in searching out the right gift for each person. He was probably one of the few adults left who still enjoyed Christmas—filling stockings for the children on Christmas Eve was one of his great delights, and if they didn't bulge enough to suit him, he would go around the house finding more Scotch tape, or jars of nuts, or whatever, until the stockings were so heavy they could barely be hung.

Now that he was bedridden, he still thought about presents, and as various family birthdays came and went Limey wanted to know what I was going to get, wanted to discuss it with me, and usually ended up telling me what to buy. When our wedding anniversary came around, Limey was very upset because he couldn't, as he always had, go out and buy me something, and in fact he had Jimmy and his wife select a pair of earrings for me to match a necklace he had gotten me the year before. That he remembered and was concerned with this, in spite of all his body involvement and his constant frustration, was the most precious gift of all.

However, I still was ready to borrow money if it became necessary to pay more than I had planned in order to get someone to come in to work. People go into debt to buy cars and boats and furniture and television sets, yet I have known those same people to consider it too much of an extravagance to borrow to hire help when they desperately need it to save themselves. I didn't think that way. I wasn't eager to go into debt, but it wouldn't be the end of the world—the possibility of my collapsing was the scary one, so I had to hang on to my sanity and health for dear life.

Luckily, though, I didn't have to borrow, because I found Millie. Millie was a widow in her early fifties who had nursed her own husband through a long illness. She didn't live far away, she had her own car, and she wanted to work. Millie was a nice person with a lot of problems. She was a nervous woman and she had a history of starting out first-rate with several jobs and then losing them because she petered out. I soon discovered that Millie had a memory like a sieve, and that even when I wrote everything out for her, it did not necessarily mean that she would follow instructions.

So I had to make compromises. I made two decisions during Millie's first week. One was that I could not make a perfect world for Limey. If I told her to give him Jell-O for lunch (his main meal) and she gave him applesauce instead, it wasn't worth fussing about. He might have a loose bowel movement, but that was less important than getting Millie into a nervous state. My top priority was to make Millie feel that she was indispensable and, with all her imperfections, she was. Millie did get gratification out of what she was doing, and I tried every way I knew to help her do that.

My other decision was to vow not to get sucked into arguments with Limey. If there were days when he didn't want to get into the wheelchair, I was not going to fight about it. The Battle of the Wheelchair was a pretty constant war, but when it got too much for me I let him win.

The first time that I persuaded Millie to help me get Limey into the wheelchair broke the tension. Understandably she was nervous, and Limey was too. We swung him around to a sitting position on the bed, and we sat there, one on each side of him, while I tried to humor Limey's routine patter and to assure Millie that it didn't take any strength or size to do the job. "Why, I've seen tiny girls in the nursing home do this," I told Millie. "I'm no professional and I haven't had any trouble so long as there are two of us." Millie's face got red when she was nervous, and it was flaming now. She was clutching Limey's arm with a viselike hold that fortunately he couldn't feel. "All right, let's go," I said.

We lifted Limey from the bed and were about to swing his buttocks onto the seat of the wheelchair when it started to slide away from him. Maybe Millie had accidentally kicked the brake with her foot. I don't know exactly what happened, except that slowly, inevitably, Limey slid to the floor. The expression on Limey's face hardly changed; he looked up at us from the floor with calm resignation, as if to say "What else could be expected?" After a few seconds of horrified exclamations, and assuring ourselves that Limey wasn't hurt, a low giggle escaped from Millie. That was all I needed to start me off, and in a minute the three of us were laughing quite uncontrollably. It was a good laugh, but we still had to face the problem of how to get Limey up. I put a pillow under his head while we tried to figure out how to do it. Limey was dead weight and it didn't seem likely that we could lift him.

"I could stay here," Limey said quite cheerfully, eyeing the wheelchair balefully. "It's better than that damn chair."

"You're a good sport, but I don't think this floor is the best place for you," I told him.

Millie and I each took an arm, and we got him up to a sitting position, and then, somehow, we managed to get him up on his half-bent, very wobbly legs, and onto the now carefully braked chair. With that episode, Millie endeared herself to me. She was able to laugh, and she didn't panic. Those qualities were worth a lot of forgetfulness.

So we embarked on something that resembled a

routine. There were interruptions—the physical therapist arriving once a week, the visiting nurse once a week, and the days when Millie seemed quite out of it. But I worked, and I somehow managed to finish the book I had planned to write in Florida.

Yet I knew that I was living on the edge of a crisis. Each day I didn't know what that day would bring, and I woke up every morning with a tremendous apprehension. What if something happened to Limey and he died? Often I went into his room at night, even when he didn't call me, to make sure he was alive. And my fear was equally great that he could go on this way for years, or very possibly get worse, and still go on for years. I could see no happy ending to this story.

And yet the days were not completely downbeat. My friends were feeling sorry for me, and, believe me, I had times of terrible despair, but as wise Lillian Hellman says in her book *Scoundrel Time,* "change, loss, an altered life is only a danger when you become devoted to disaster." Determinedly I sought divertissements. That was all life had to offer me, I figured, as relief from Limey's pain and my own. I needed the warmth of close friends and especially those couples who were leading normal, active lives. I needed to be reminded of a world in which people went on vacations, went to theaters and movies, and had dinner parties. I went out in the evenings when I could get someone, usually one of the young people in town, to stay with Limey and found the experience strange. I was in a gray world where I was neither a widow nor a wife; I was alone but I was still part of a union. I think some friends expected me to feel guilty about going out, but I didn't, perhaps because I knew that any time I spent away from home was a cosmetic, a surface experience, like the amusement of a new eye shadow when you knew the dark lines underneath were still there.

I treasured the quiet times I had with Limey alone, and I like to feel that he did too, as he seemed more himself then, quieter, as if he were able to rest more comfortably. I watched the six o'clock news with him, I read to him, and sometimes if there was an interesting evening show on TV we watched it together. I got the "Talking Records" for him through our public library, but Limey did not like them. He complained that "the voices are all flat, spoken in a monotone," and he found them boring.

Also, I needed time to be by myself. I wasn't used to having people in the house all the time. I had had my house to myself for work, for puttering, for cooking, for just sitting. Almost every day I took Jo for long walks in our woods, across the fields, and on our dirt roads. These walks became very precious and I think helped me considerably. We go through life thinking we will never die, and yet every year we are surrounded by the life-death cycle of nature. But still we are impervious, we each think we are immortal. I began to think that it is this gargantuan misconception that has made our culture so careless with the quality of life. Limey was not having a good life. He was, in fact, having a terrible life. But the irony, the both tragic and remarkable irony, was that he was making a contribution to my life that was as valuable as anything he had given me in the past. I was learning to be selective, developing a discrimination that was in a good measure his. He had no time or energy to be bothered with silly people. When I asked him if he wanted to see so-and-so he would bluntly say yes or no, and it was easy to understand why. I found myself agreeing with him, instead of, as in the past, wasting time with some people who meant very little to either of us. When I went for my walks I noticed for the first time the plants and the wild-flowers, the way he always had. Now, *now* I was learning his values, adding them to my own. This tragic, crippled man, without ever knowing it, was making me grow. Neither Limey nor I had ever been religious, and we were not now turning to religion to find comfort as many people do. But Limey's great respect for nature, which included a philosophical view of the life-death cycle, along with my own strong sense of life and a kind of simple trust in man's ability to endure, made me feel that somehow or other "things would work themselves out." Each day that we were able to hang on, avoid a new disaster or setback, manage a laugh or two, exchange affection, was in itself making our life work.

This fine, philosophical gold, however, was struck only on good days. For a great deal of the time it was frustrating, sad, and sometimes angry digging. Outside of Millie's absentmindedness, her one big flaw was talking what Limey called "baby talk." "Dearie, will you raise your leg for me?"

"If I can raise my leg, it will not be for you, it will be for myself," Limey would answer in no uncertain terms.

Or "Come on, love, take a spoon of this for me," in the

tone of a mother coaxing an infant. If Limey could, I
think he might have thrown the bowl of soup or cereal at
her.

Once, when he was well fastened in his wheelchair, he
complained that he felt he was falling, as he often did,
and Millie said, "It only feels that way."

"Of course it only feels that way," Limey said, outraged
by the absurdity of her logic, and I was thankful that he
waited until she was out of earshot to say, "That woman
is an idiot." Limey was always correcting her English.
When he said, "Nothing can be very unique," she looked
perplexed. "But it is," she insisted. "I've never seen more
than half a dozen double-yolk eggs like this. They are
very unique." But in a way he was fond of her, and on the
whole they got along well.

One of our big problems was taking care of his backside. It was almost impossible for his rear end not to become tender and sore, sometimes with open wounds, in
spite of the constant care he got. I never minded taking
care of Limey's body. Nothing was ever offensive to me,
as nothing is offensive in intimacy with someone you love.
But I could not bear his crying. "Hila wants me to be a
stoic," Limey dictated into his tape recorder. "She wants
me to be brave and heroic and I am not." His words made
me weep. I did not want him to be heroic, but I could not
bear his crying. Sometimes he cried like an infant when
he had to be cleaned, and I could never get myself to tell
him how much it pained me to hear him cry—he was as
unabashed about crying when he was hurt as he was
about his incontinence. I was the one afraid to burst into

tears. So, my God, he believed I wanted him to be brave. Bravery, dignity . . . keep your chin up . . . neither Limey nor I had much use for bravery. Courage, yes, but courage has little to do with crying or not crying. Maybe it takes courage to cry . . . yet I did not want to cry in front of Limey and I felt absolutely distraught when he cried, although God knows he had reason and I didn't give a damn about his being brave. It was just so terribly, terribly sad.

The quality of life has become a popular phrase, and yet we still all talk about it as something for the future. But when you feel there is no future that is bright, when you are down at the bottom, hanging on, then you begin to examine the quality of your life in the here and now. My way of doing it was to sit up and take notice, to be more aware of what I can only call basic values: to distinguish between givers and takers, to want amusement but not crap, to be more protective of my time, not to say yes when I meant no, and perhaps most of all to take each day as it came and not to get myself into a morbid depression thinking about what was going to happen. "What are you going to do?" was a question I was no longer willing to discuss. Dammit, I was doing it, day by day, and when the future came it would be another day that would be faced when it arrived.

A new day came sooner than I expected. It came by way of the physical therapist around a month after Limey was home. "I think Mr. Colman should get more therapy than he's getting here," she said. "Have you thought about putting him in a rehabilitation center?" She mentioned a well-known institution in Westchester County.

"He was supposed to have been in one when he was in the nursing home, but it really wasn't what he needed," I said.

"This place is a hospital, not a nursing home, and the people there are specialists in helping stroke patients. I think you should look into it. Ask your doctor what he thinks. I've never been there but I've been told it's a fabulous place."

While she was still in the house I called the neurologist in New York and he said, "Sure, I have no objection. It's a good idea, but I doubt you can get him in there. It's certainly worth trying."

I asked Limey how he felt about it, should he get in, and he was agreeable. "I don't want to go to a nursing home, though," he said.

"It's a hospital. I imagine a place like the Rusk Institute in New York. I'll find out."

After several telephone calls I was finally connected with a doctor at the hospital who told me that he accepted no patient who had had a stroke more than four weeks previous, without an evaluation. "We have a limited number of beds," he said crisply, "and we keep a patient here on an average of from six to eight weeks. If you want to bring your husband in for an evaluation, there is no guarantee that he will be admitted. You can call my secretary for an appointment if you decide to come."

"I'd have to bring him in an ambulance. How long would he be there?"

"Perhaps an hour or two. You'd have to keep the ambulance to take him home."

"Yes, I see that. It would be very expensive."

"It's up to you," he said curtly.

"Yes, I know. I'll think about it. Thank you."

I didn't think about it for long. My first three-minute reaction, however, was one of rage. Why in hell didn't someone tell me to send him there directly from the New York hospital four weeks after his stroke? Obviously that was when he would have been the best candidate for help. Later our neurologist said that he had mentioned it, but mentioning it had not been enough. I made myself calm down and reviewed in my mind all the reasons we had chosen the place in Connecticut: the promise of rehabilitation, good surroundings, near the children, the notion that in our resident state we could get financial assistance (false) . . . I will never know if it would have made any difference, but I did know that thinking about what I might have done was a useless, wasteful line of breast-beating. I had to believe that I had done what I thought best, and what seemed best at the time, and the only thing to do now was to take the next step. And I did.

I set up an appointment and made arrangements with the ambulance service to take us down and wait to bring us home. So, several days later, Limey and I went for another ambulance ride. We came to an impressive institution, with extensive, magnificently kept lawns and trees, and with me pushing Limey on a stretcher were directed to a Dr. Stern's office. Dr. Stern, however, was occupied, and we waited in a reception room outside his office.

Limey promptly fell asleep. This made me extremely nervous. My God, I thought, after all this, he'll be sound asleep when we are to see the doctor, and, knowing the routine by now, Limey will never be able to answer the questions that will be thrown at him. I kept nudging him to wake up, and he'd half open his eyes sleepily and then go right off again. The hour wait seemed interminable.

At last the secretary told us that Dr. Stern was ready to see us. We were greeted by a young bearded man in a white coat who looked like a hundred other doctors. The first thing he did was to be annoyed that Limey was on a stretcher instead of in a wheelchair and he quickly got some orderlies to remedy that. Limey still seemed very drowsy, and continued to appear sleepy throughout the quick examination of his arms and legs and the taking of his history.

"Does he always hold his head to the side like that?" Dr. Stern asked.

"More or less," I told him. "More when he's tired." I was thinking I'd wasted a lot of time, energy, and money coming down to this place.

I was sure of it when Dr. Stern started firing his questions at Limey. All I could think of was when I'd taken our sons for interviews to get into prep school and to various colleges and the nervous tension of knowing damn well that they were not doing their best. "Who was Calvin Coolidge?" Limey barely opened his eyes when he answered, "Vice-President to Harding and became President when Harding died. Then I think he served a full term 1924–28."

The next was a complicated mathematical question that I couldn't answer at all. In a bored voice, Limey gave the correct answer in a few seconds. Then there were a series of proverbs that required philosophical answers, which Limey gave in the same half-sleepy way. By this time I suspect I was grinning like a smug mama.

Dr. Stern looked at me. "This man has a mind."

"I know," I said. The bored expression on Limey's face didn't change.

Dr. Stern was obviously impressed. I suppose a good many stroke patients whom he saw with Limey's encompassing physical disabilities had more impairment of their mental faculties than Limey did. But none of the doctors seemed to take into consideration that Limey had a better than average brain to start with.

"I don't know what to say. I'm really in a dilemma." The good doctor looked distraught. "It is against my principle to admit anyone to my ward who has had a stroke more than four weeks before. That is how I work, and we only have limited beds." He was telling me everything he had told me on the phone. "But this man has a mind. I would really like to help him, and I think we can. I don't know what to do. I honestly don't know . . ."

I sat without saying a word. Some blessed instinct told me not to beg, not to start beseeching. I could see on Dr. Stern's face that he was truly struggling to come to a decision, and he would not welcome any interference in making up his mind. I was quiet, but my heart was beating like a sledgehammer. I was fastened on to the words "I think we can help him." I am not religious, but I think I may have prayed silently.

Finally Dr. Stern looked across his desk at me. "All right. Out of compassion for this man, and for you, I will admit him. It is terrible to see a man with a good, alert mind suffer as he is. You must promise me one thing. When it is time for him to be discharged I don't want you to come begging me to keep him on. I told you, an average stay in my ward is six to eight weeks. You won't be told overnight, you'll get notice. But when it's time for him to go, he goes."

"I understand. You don't have to worry about it. I very much appreciate what you are doing. Thank you."

"See my secretary, she will make the arrangements. There will be some wait for a bed, I don't know how long. Maybe a week or two, I don't know."

I thanked him again and wheeled Limey out. I wished I had been able to throw my arms around that doctor. He had just handed a drowning couple a lifeline. My elation knew no bounds. That place seemed so exactly right, there was a professionalism I had not seen before, and I trusted Dr. Stern. He had a combination of dedication and compassion. The patients I saw in the halls in their wheelchairs all seemed to be going somewhere, they weren't just sitting, and they didn't look beaten down. They looked like people who were going to get well, or at least better than when they had come in. You saw no one in pajamas or robes. Everyone was dressed, people were

talking and laughing, nurses and orderlies were joking
with each other.

Dr. Stern's secretary was truly surprised. "Is he really
admitted? He never does that. You're very lucky."

"I know." I was grinning from ear to ear.

"You'll have to go around and see the woman in charge
of admissions. She'll need some information from you
and she's the one who will let you know when a bed is
available."

"Do you have an idea how long that might be?"

The young woman shook her head. "A few weeks
probably."

When we got home I called everyone to tell them the
good news. I felt that our luck was changing. After all,
the months since Limey had had his stroke hadn't been
wasted. He'd had therapy, we had been doing the exercises faithfully at home twice a day (every day, not skip-
ping weekends), and God knows he was considerably
better than the day I had first seen him in the hospital in
New York when I'd come up from Florida. He'd been
flat on his back then, being fed through a tube. Now he
was up in his wheelchair several hours a day, he was able
to feed himself with some success, he was using his tape
recorder, able to watch television—there *was* a difference.
And I felt very good about the rehabilitation center. If
any place was going to be able to help him, this was it.
Also I felt good about myself. I knew that, whatever happened, I was leaving no stone unturned. So far I had not

fallen apart and had somehow summoned up the energy to make another move. It would have been easy to rationalize not bothering to take Limey on a day's ambulance journey, when the question of his admittance had been so iffy. But even if he was going to be turned down, I was positive that we had to take the chance.

Now we were in a waiting period again. One of my concerns was losing the people working for us. Would the VNA have an aide available when we came back? And what about Millie? With all her faults, I didn't want to lose her. We talked about it, and since she had not been working for some time before she came to us, she said that she didn't mind staying home until Limey came back again. I could only hope that she meant it.

I hated waiting to hear. Each morning I thought, they *have* to call today. Every time the phone rang I jumped to reach it. I felt that every day was a day lost for Limey, and I was nagged by the thought that if a bed didn't materialize soon Dr. Stern would change his mind and say it was too late. Often I thought of all the times over the years I'd waited for phone calls. Calls from lovers, calls from Limey, calls from our sons, calls from doctors, calls from schools . . . I had never learned to forget about waiting to hear, and now waiting for this call seemed to overshadow all the others. It occurred to me that whether Limey was willing to fight for his life or not, I was, and I was fighting for it every minute of the day.

Part Three

On the Friday afternoon of Memorial Day weekend, the call came. "Bring Mr. Colman down on Sunday. We'd like him here before two o'clock."

"On this holiday weekend?"

"Sunday before two."

Just the day before, I had said to Limey, "I'm going to forget about the phone if we don't hear today. I'm sure we won't hear over this weekend, so I can relax until Monday."

But I wasn't sorry the call had come. That is, not until I tried getting an ambulance for that Sunday. Our Volunteer Fire Department's ambulance could not go out of town on a holiday because there was no backup in the area. This, I discovered, was also true of all the surrounding towns, for the same reason. Understandably, no one was willing to leave his own town uncovered for likely

holiday emergencies. Why did they want him to come
this Sunday of all times! It seemed as if everything, every
single step, was an uphill battle. Nothing was easy, nothing was designed for the individual—we were the victims
of a relentless bureaucracy. Limey had to leave the hospital (ready or not) because they could not keep him any
longer; Limey had to leave the nursing home because he
was not progressing rapidly enough to suit Medicare;
Limey has to come to the rehabilitation center on this day
at this hour because they say so . . . why the devil
couldn't he go there on Monday morning? No, we would
lose the bed. I felt part of a parade where, if I fell down,
no one would pick me up. I had to keep marching. So I
spent Saturday on the telephone and finally found a com-
mercial ambulance service that, for a considerable sum,
would pick us up on Sunday morning and take us to
Westchester. (Eventually I got back part of the ambulance cost from Medicare.)

Limey was nervous about another move. A good deal of
my anger was caused by the fact that I should have been,
I wanted to be, with Limey that Saturday instead of hanging on the phone trying to get a damned ambulance. He
needed me, and I suddenly realized, in the midst of my
excitement about his getting into the rehab center, that I
was going to miss him. The visiting nurse and the therapist, both of whom had been very pleased that Limey had
been admitted, had said, "It will be a good rest for you."
They were closer to and more aware of the daily situation
in our household than anyone else, and I often felt and
appreciated their warm empathy and concern for me. I

am not an overly modest woman, but I did not feel heroic. I was grateful that I had the strength and the energy to do what had to be done, but no one knew my subjective feelings. I have figured out that I was in love with two people: the Limey that was, and when flashes of his humor and wit, his discernment, came through I was ecstatic; and this crippled, garrulous, helpless, difficult man that he had now become. The fact that he was a burden (God knows I cannot minimize that), and that we could not have the closeness in any way that we had had, did not turn me away from him. I suppose the fact that he was so dependent on me, the way a child is on his parents, played a part in my feelings. We no longer had the same two-way, interdependent relationship, and yet so many times in the course of the day, working in my study, or taking a break and going in to have a visit with Limey, I felt so glad that he was here. I could see him, talk to him, touch him. And every day we had was precious. The future was too scary. Sometimes I looked at other couples who were going through the usual squabbling, a wife's frustration and tears, a husband's bewilderment and anger, and I thought, you fools, you don't know, you just don't know. But no one knows. No one could have stopped Limey and me from fighting when he was well, but the big thing was, I found that it didn't matter. What mattered was not whether we had been gentle and tender or angry and harsh (we had been all of those things) but that we still reacted to each other so totally, each providing feedback for the other.

The very quality that had made Limey not an easy man

to live with also made him interesting: his intensity. He felt strongly about everything, and expressed his point of view in absolutes—even his indifference was a positive statement. There was no mistaking the fact that there was another personality in the house, that I had someone to contend with; yet for all his strong reactions, he was a gentle person. In some ways my independence had not been good for Limey, although he never tried to hold me back. Limey liked to take care of people—he diapered babies and tended the boys' and our various animals' wounds, and he cooked for me and waited on me magnificently whenever I was tired or not feeling well, or just plain lazy. I think Limey was fooled by my so-called independence—because I could go to Europe by myself, or earn money, and had a few old friends separate from those we had together, he thought I did not need him. What he did not know, because he had not been there to see, was that before I lived with Limey I had been a floundering person. Yes, I had been young then, but Limey had *character,* a good old-fashioned word, and if I stood up well during his illness it was because he had given me some of that, and I don't think he ever knew how much I depended on his character for my guidelines. You could not do anything shoddy with Limey looking on, whether it was accepting too much change from a storekeeper, entertaining a phony twice, or buying something obviously tacky. In Mexico, where it was the common practice, Limey refused to bargain. If he wanted something, he paid what was asked and was contemptuous of doing business any other way. But to think now about my dependence on Limey was not a safe path to pursue—it could lead too easily to tears. There had been times when I thought, my God, I cannot go on living with this man, he is impossible, he has a temper, he is too much of a perfectionist, I do not need someone with such standards that neither he nor anyone else can live up to them—for all his tenderness and love, he can cut someone down like no one I ever knew. But I knew I never could or would leave him because dependence is a part of any love, emotional dependence. Yes, I was dependent on Limey.

I think most of us cannot believe how much everything we say and do affects our partner. Everyone thinks that only he is vulnerable and has no idea at all of his own power to affect someone else. It is a perverse kind of put-down of one's self, this forgetting that when you are living with someone, a husband or wife, a lover, your children, there is always an audience there responding.

During his illness Limey, I am sure, had little or no idea of how his every mood or tiny change affected me. And that was what I would miss, the good and the bad, when he went away again. An editor wrote to me recently, "You are a complicated lady . . ." and I thought, how simple, down to basics, the most complicated person can become. Limey needed only to greet me in the morning saying, "I'm hungry, and please turn on the 'Today' show," to brighten my life. My reasoning was simple: when a man's hungry he's not dying, and if he wants to look at something in the world outside of his discomfort, his spirit is healthy too. And I could become ecstatic if, when watching the show, he uttered one of his on-target caustic remarks about some fellow who didn't know what he was talking about, or a pretty woman who didn't have to talk, or expressed his admiration for a gallant under-dog. By the same token, he could send me into despair when he rambled on about his past, repeating things he had said a hundred times, and, believe it or not, get me into a wild, crazy jealousy when he talked about his first wife, who had been dead for over forty years.

"I'm cleaning your ass and you're talking about a woman who's been dead for nearly half a century," I yelled at him once.

Limey was utterly surprised. "What's one got to do with the other?" he asked mildly.

"Nothing," I said tersely. "Absolutely nothing." But of course it had everything to do with it, and it didn't take freshman psychology to figure out that I was indulging in a foolish bit of fanciful drama: Stoic, middle-aged Hila with a shiny nose and uncombed hair diligently doing the messy work while Himself nostalgically grieved for a beautiful young woman in her twenties who died in the youth's tender arms. Who needed it?

But maybe I did need it. I was never ready to put my emotions on the back of the stove, to accept the helpless man that fate had handed me and to treat him as such. I happen to believe that it had to be good for Limey too, to have a wife who did not treat him as if he were already dead, but who still got angry and jealous, who was not robbing him of the one power he had left, the power to arouse my feelings. How awful if I had been only compassionate and solicitous—hell, he could get that from a nurse, but I was still his wife, a complicated and emotional woman who did not whisper in soft sickroom tones, and he was still my husband, who, although he could not turn himself over in bed, could very much get a rise out of me.

Our son Jimmy said the other day, "We should not have screamed at Dad that weekend he came home from the nursing home." He was ashamed. I feel some shame too, the normal shame of losing one's temper, and yet I am not really sorry, because I was hanging on, as I continued to hang on, to all the threads of life, as ephemeral and as strong as a spider's web, that had been spun between Limey and me.

On Sunday morning at ten o'clock the ambulance arrived. Once again Limey was carried out on a stretcher, but this time I knew enough to bring along a suitcase of clothes, and we also brought our borrowed wheelchair. "Bring my cane," Limey said. "I want my cane." Limey's insistence on his cane broke my heart. Somewhere this man, who so often said he was tortured and begged to die, somewhere he still embraced a glimmer of hope that he would get himself out of bed and walk again. His cry for his cane was not one of desolation, he commanded with a firm voice, and I marveled at both the tenacity of life and the protective warmth of self-delusion.

This time an attendant sat with Limey and I rode with Jimmy in my car. It was an exciting ride. Jimmy loved keeping a fast pace behind the ambulance, cutting through the traffic, breaking the fifty-five-mile-an-hour speed limit without fear of getting a ticket. I felt good that Sunday, full of hope and with a peaceful sense that we were doing what was best and right. I still feel that way.

Limey was taken to a large room that he would share with one other male patient. The room was bright and sunny and looked out on a greenhouse and gardens (which he could not see), and each bed had a color television set, hung from the ceiling and easily visible to the patient reclining in bed. Jimmy was impressed, as I had been, with the physical setup of the place and with the general atmosphere. When a handsome, young, dark-skinned woman came in to greet Limey and to take his history, we were even more impressed.

Besides the routine questions about his illness and his paralysis, she asked him many personal questions about his thoughts, his interests, the things he had liked to do when he was well, what kind of work he had done. "We are going to be working together," she said, "and I want to know as much about you as I possibly can." She spoke in a sober and strong way. "You are going to have to work hard here. Sometimes you are going to be in pain—and it is not because we want to hurt you, believe me. We are here to help you in every way we can, but you are the one who has to do the work, and to work hard." She emphasized that point strongly.

"Well, how do you feel about it?" I asked Limey after she had left.

"I think it's going to be all right," he said.

"I'm glad you're here. I think they can help you."

"We'll see," Limey said, and his eyes looked off into the distance, and then closed wearily.

Jimmy and I stayed with him awhile and then we left him. Downstairs, in an open area with tables and umbrellas, it looked like there was a party going on. There were several patients in wheelchairs, and a young man with a leg missing was playing a guitar for a group of young friends gathered around him. They had evidently sent out for Chinese food and were eating the various dishes out of cardboard cartons and having a rousing time. Jimmy and I left in high spirits. There was nothing depressing about this place—it was lively and active: people came here to get better.

I was not unhappy when I came home. It was strange not having Limey there, and all the people who came and went, but when someone called and asked if I wanted to go out to dinner and a movie, it was rather nice not to have to worry about getting someone to stay with Limey. The nurse and the therapist had been right. I hadn't realized under what a strain I had been operating, and this was a respite for me. The main thing, though, was the knowledge I kept hugging to myself, that while I was home, writing, even having some fun, a really dedicated and top-notch team was working for Limey. We were not standing still.

My plan was to visit Limey twice during the week, going down late in the afternoon after I had gotten in a day's work, and spending one day over the weekend with him. The first week nothing much happened. There was a bulletin board up near the nurses' desk, and I noticed that most of the other patients had several appointments during the day, but Limey had only one, to go down to physical therapy. I asked the head nurse why.

"He has to get acclimated," she told me. "He said he's not interested in group discussion, and we will start his occupational therapy next week."

"You have to understand my husband," I said. "Don't pay too much attention to his first negative reaction. Of course he'll say he doesn't care about group discussion—the name would put him off. But I think if you took him to it, he might become interested. I'd try it."

"Thank you for telling me. We have to get to know him too." She looked at me with sympathetic eyes. "Don't expect miracles here. Your husband has a lot of problems."

"I know that. My goals are very limited. I am hoping you people may be able to get him to sit on a toilet, or a pot-chair next to the bed. I hope that he can learn to feed himself better than he does, and very important, that you can get him interested in the outside world again. His mind is good but it's hard to get his attention away from his problems."

"I know. Can you suggest anything?"

"He likes to watch the news. You could have someone turn on the 'Today' show in the morning and the six o'clock news in the evening. I see a sign next to his bed that you're not supposed to plug anything in—I suppose they don't want to blow fuses—but if I could bring down his tape recorder, he might use it."

"That would be good. We can plug that in—it's part of his therapy."

I liked her. She was open and warm and friendly. Actually I liked all of the staff I had met so far. Especially one very young man (I don't think he was more than twenty-one or twenty-two) who talked with Limey about books and asked me to bring down some of Limey's poetry for him and the chaplain to read. The poems filled two notebooks, and I think they helped them to know Limey better. The following is one that I particularly like:

"Watching and Wondering"

We walked and wandered in the woods and fields and swamps
    together
watching and wondering
the blacksnake gliding on the hot stone wall
the birthday cakes of bluets and the small white spiral orchid
    in the pasture
Hepaticas deep in the shade—our first; to make us gasp and
    catch our breaths
Pleurotus by the bushel in the swamp
morels and water cress in the old orchard and the brook

And in our room, six captive turtles
heads held high
clumped thunderous thunderous
clockwise

along the walls
Waiting the coming storm

The next week Louis Colman's calendar had more appointments scheduled. He had the usual ones for physical and occupational therapy, one to go to the greenhouse, one for group discussion, and, much to my surprise, one for Sunday services. "Did you really go to the chapel?" I asked my anticlerical husband. Limey was never against religion, but he had never gotten over his youthful rebellion against organized churchgoing.

"Yes, I did. The chaplain is a very interesting man. He's the only person around here to talk to. He wants to meet you."

"I'd be delighted to meet him."

On a later visit I did meet the chaplain, and I could understand why Limey had taken to him. He was an interesting, well-read, knowledgeable, unpretentious man. He told me that he and Limey had great discussions about such things as the difference between pride and vanity, jealousy and envy, biblical stories, and the philosophy of religion.

But my visits were far from all upbeat. Like an anxious researcher examining a specimen through a microscope, I kept looking for improvements, sometimes, I suspect, making them up if I didn't find them. It was so agonizingly slow, whatever changes there were were almost imperceptible. I only saw Dr. Stern when I caught him in the halls. "We're making some progress," he said on the run. "He's moving his right side better. He can tolerate the wheelchair longer than he did. It's very slow, I admit, it's very slow . . . Bring your family down, take him outside, have some picnics . . ."

Picnics . . . that was a lovely idea, and we did it. I had taken advantage of my time at home to have my grand-children come to visit in pairs, and I had taken the older ones down to see Limey. Then we arranged for all of us, Jon and Wanda and their five, and Jimmy and Joyce and their little one, to have a Sunday picnic with Limey. I made huge quantities of barbecued chicken and salads, we brought wine and fresh rolls and fruit and cookies, and we descended upon the hospital. We wheeled Limey out to a roofed but open colonnade overlooking a great lawn and garden, and we had our picnic. It was a poi-gnant affair. Limey was with us, but not with us. I think he enjoyed it, he enjoyed his sons and the children, yet every few minutes he asked to be pulled up on the chair, he asked to have his eyes wiped—we could not really get him involved with the family. He tired quickly, and Jonny soon had to take him back to his room. He seemed grateful to get back into bed. However, he did talk about it afterward, and I know it meant something to him. We did it a second time with about the same results.

And so the weeks went by. I found myself going through the same seesaw of emotions, hoping, hoping, driving to the hospital telling myself that this day there will be a breakthrough, today there will be a jump for-ward that I will see, an improvement that will be unmis-takable. I would go through the long driveway, park the car, go inside and up in the elevator with my heart beating nervously. I don't know what I expected to find. I suppose some manifestation of the old Limey who had always greeted me when I came home, whose face lit up as he took my bundles from me while he said, "No one called. The phone never rings when you are not home," then grinned with satisfaction and annoyance when the phone would ring at precisely that moment. "See, I told you, they know you're home."

No, it wouldn't be the same Limey, but perhaps some gesture, some reminder of that man who had responded so totally to love and warmth. I guess that was the big difference: I was still responding, but he wasn't. Perhaps that's not fair. While clearly he was wrapped up in the awful problems he had to deal with, I cannot say that he did not feel emotions, but his responses were so faint, so swathed in his own agony, it was difficult to know if he was able to get any pleasure out of anything or anyone. I like to think that he did, and I always went on the assumption that he welcomed my visits and those of the other people who came to see him, that he did get some enjoyment out of some of our conversations and the few delicacies he would eat. While he talked about food, and he dictated some thoughts on food, he was really not interested in eating anymore. The effort of feeding himself, he said, was tiring, but even when he was fed he was not interested and said that he had lost his sense of taste.

Inevitably the day came when the social worker called and said that she wanted to make an appointment to see me. Oh Lord, I thought, do I have to go through that again? At the time I was having my fill of what I classi-

fied as "unpleasant business arrangements." During one
of my frequent four o'clock in the morning awakenings, I
had suddenly panicked at the thought of what would
happen to Limey if something happened to me. I was his
lifeline—and what if I got hit by a truck? The thought
kept me from settling back to sleep. It was conceivable
that he could outlive me.

The next day I made a proposal to Limey. It was a
hard, but I believe, practical decision, and he agreed
wholeheartedly. Whatever Limey and I had, our house
and savings, we owned jointly, and in our wills we had
left everything to each other. I suggested we change that.
I wanted to put everything in my name and to leave what
there was to be equally divided between our two sons. My
thinking was that obviously Limey could not handle any
finances—our sons would have to handle that anyway,
and it would be simpler if they owned the house, in case it
had to be sold, and whatever was left of our savings. We
both knew there was no question about their taking care
of Limey—if he could remain home with a nurse or
housekeeper, they would see to it. If he had to go to a
nursing home, then since he would not have any funds of
his own, he could go in under Medicaid, and in that case,
frankly we preferred that our sons receive whatever benefits there were of our years of hard work rather than an
institution—and what we had wouldn't last long in a
nursing home anyway.

I have a great distaste for this sort of thing. It meant
going to see a lawyer, drawing up a new will, getting our
property and bonds transferred to my name—explaining

each document to Limey and guiding his hand in signing every paper—it was all terribly unpleasant, but when it was done I was relieved that our affairs were in some order for Limey's welfare. Still, as objective as one tries to be, the subjective factors insistently get in the way. I spilled many tears over how our life together was ending up, and although our lack of material assets had been more conspicuous than our gains, each acquisition had held the promise of an enjoyable old age: we would do some traveling, we would have a large garden, read the books we hadn't had time for, clean out our woods of dead brush and trees . . .

During the five years since Limey's first stroke he had been at home, and we had become more dependent on each other than ever before. Dependent in a good way, sharing our thoughts, planning our trips, discussing our writing and what we were each reading, planning our meals, going marketing, enjoying our kids, and fighting less. I had thought, how nice that we were going to have a good old age together, not be a cantankerous pair who got on each other's nerves. That first stroke of Limey's had relieved him of the tensions of a daily job, and actually we worried less about money than we had before. Our income was pretty well fixed: he had his social security and small pension and I knew more or less what I could count on from my books, and what we got from our small savings, and that was that. Foolishly, I suppose, I had never thought about Limey having a second stroke. I had thought our life would just go on its rather even way indefinitely. We had not planned for what had happened, and when I had written the one will in my life I had never thought I would write another.

At any rate, in the midst of all this the call from the social worker came and I went down to see her. She was a less uptight woman than the other social workers I had encountered, but the same old question was posed: "What are you going to do when Mr. Colman leaves here?"

"Take him home," I told her.

"How will you manage? Do you have any help lined up?"

"We managed before, and we'll do it again. I hope to get a nurse's aide from the VNA, and to get the same woman who worked for us before."

She looked at me with the same kind of eyes I'd seen so often before: an expression of sympathy, skepticism, and enough pity to make me feel teary and uncomfortable. Nothing could set me off weeping as quickly as pity.

"If you change your mind, get in touch with me. Perhaps I can help find a suitable nursing home."

"They're all too expensive. Besides, I don't like them that much."

She shook her head sadly. "It's going to be very hard to care for him at home."

"I guess he hasn't improved very much, has he?"

Her eyes told me the answer, which, of course, I already knew. "Everyone worked very hard for him."

I knew the interview meant that Limey was going to be discharged in the near future. "There's no rush," she said. "Whenever you are ready he can go. In the meantime I

want to set up appointments with the physical and occupational therapists. And it would be a good idea to bring
the woman down with you who will be taking care of
him. She can see the whole routine."

I went outside to a magnificent, bright, sunny day and
hated it. Gloomy rain and a dull gray sky would have
suited me better. I used to think of myself as a sun person,
and now I wondered if I would ever truly enjoy anything
again. At that point I couldn't even muster up any anger.
I just felt beat—something like having put every cent you
owned on a horse race and losing. You win some, you lose
some. But I could not be that philosophical. I had been
betting on our life. (I never thought of it as Limey's life
alone. Maybe that is why I fought so hard—I was fighting
for my own life too.)

At home I did all the things that I had to do. I alerted
Millie. I called up the VNA and told them I would need a
nurse's aide again soon. I went down to New York to
take care of some business. I went up to Cambridge to see
my kids—I felt pushed to crowd in as much as possible
before I entered a long siege, much as if I were going to
prison.

It was a bad time and a bad mood. However, I also
covered myself as much as possible for the future. When I
learned that my nurse's aide this time would come for the
morning hours from eight to noon, I hired Millie to come
from noon to six, every weekday except Thursday, which
she would have off as well as Sunday, and to give me all
day on Saturday. Then I also proceeded to find a young

woman with some nursing background to come in on Sundays. I was not going to go through frantic weekends again.

This was going to be expensive. But, with Medicare paying for the nurse's aide, it still came to only about half of what a nursing home would be. I felt it was my only salvation and that somehow or other I would manage. What fascinates me is the confidence I had that I would manage, and that if the future turned out otherwise, I would find some other solution. Obviously, in the seven months since Limey had become so ill, I had learned something. The very fact that I, who had done a considerable amount of floundering in my life, who had been dependent emotionally and in making decisions on other people, had been able to find solutions to our problems gave me a new outlook. "Oh well," I can hear some voices say, "you had a profession, you could work, and you had the money." Yes, I have a profession, but my work requires a very special kind of concentration, a freedom from distraction, and an emotional equanimity, none of which, believe me, did I have during that period. Nor did we ever have an income that by any stretch of the imagination could be considered high—our income was very middle-class and, with inflation, pretty low on that scale. I am emphasizing all this, not to heap praise upon myself, but to point out that it can be done. If I could take care of Limey at home, then it is a viable solution for many other people in the same predicament. Everyone was screaming nursing home at me, but it was not what I wanted—and I think that today government agencies are finding that institutional care is not proving the best for children, for handicapped people, for the retarded, for old people, or for the chronically ill, and more effort is being made to help keep those people at home.

My decision to spend a good portion of our income on help was also a result of a renewed determination to take each day as it came. I was planning for the now and the near future. If a year later I couldn't do it, I would worry about that then, and in the meantime, I hoped, I would have an arrangement at home that would not make a wreck of me.

I took Millie down to the hospital for a day. Much of what was shown us we already had learned how to do. We knew how to roll Limey to make up his bed, we knew how to move him from the bed to the wheelchair and back again. They had not succeeded in doing anything about his bowels, and had also abandoned the bedpan as well as the urinal. They used a simple sheath over his penis that was connected to a tube that emptied into a bag tied to the side of the bed. It was a practical and easy arrangement, and when Limey was discharged I was given a small supply to take home. One new procedure was putting a splint on Limey's left leg and arm at night —to keep his leg straight and to prevent his arm from curling up. When he came home he insisted that I be the one to do this for him.

We watched a very competent therapist, whom Limey had taken a great liking to, put him through his exercises in the gym. I was glad that Millie was there to watch because she had had a tendency to go through the exercises quickly and a bit on the rough side. This man emphasized, "Slowly and gently. If he says it hurts, stop." In the occupational therapy room Limey tried the typewriter but only succeeded, very painstakingly, in getting a few letters on the paper. We knew about having him pick up small objects with his fingers and had been doing that at home. They did, however, design a spoon that made it easier for him to feed himself, and I was grateful to have that.

Before Limey was to be discharged I was given an appointment to see Dr. Stern. My newfound confidence had already been considerably shaken by our day in the hospital. In everyone's face and manner I had met an unmistakable skepticism about the practicability of bringing Limey home. Sitting in Dr. Stern's office, with his eyes piercing me as if he were trying to fathom the mechanism of this strange female creature, I was not reassured. "Unfortunately your husband can live a long time," he said, looking me straight in the eye. "He's very strong. I say 'unfortunately' because he has a mind but a body that is of little use to him. He is a very unhappy man, and you and I will never know the nightmare he is living in."

He was not telling me something that I did not know, had not thought about for months, but his saying it out loud, in so many words, with a nurse and the social worker in the room, their eyes averted from me, made me choke back the tightness in my throat and blink away the tears I refused to let fall. I did not want them to feel sorry for me, because now it was anger that was burning in me. Perhaps Dr. Stern understood. "We can send men to the moon," he said, "but we cannot cure everyone who comes in here. We have failed with your husband."

I stared back at the good doctor. There was nothing for me to say. I murmured something about "Yes, we can send men to the moon, we can spend billions on missiles and weapons, but when it comes to medical research and taking care of the sick it's peanuts. . . ."

"Talk to the legislators about that," he said brusquely. "That's not the medical profession's fault."

I don't know whether if more millions had been spent on medical research my husband would have been helped, or the thousands of others hit by crippling and disabling diseases, but I do know that a burning anger was smoldering within me.

Anger was nothing new to me. But the anger I felt in Dr. Stern's office was of a different kind. It was an anger grown out of the frustration of knowing that there was no one to be angry at. I could not write a letter to my congressman and say, "Please, can you do something about my husband?"

"What are you going to do?" the doctor asked me. "I rarely recommend this, but I think for your sake and for your husband's too, he should be put into a nursing home."

A nursing home. The word "rehabilitation" had vanished. No one was pretending anymore. Now a nursing home meant a place to exist until he died. Custodial care. The words had the sound of a cemetery, a place where custodians took care of graves.

Who was he talking about? Was he talking about Limey and me?—two reasonably bright and attractive people who had gaily gotten married some thirty-odd years ago, brought up two sons, and paid off the mortgage on a house in the country, who now had two daughters-in-law they loved, six grandchildren they delighted in—two people who some seven months before had driven from Connecticut to a pleasant apartment in Florida to spend a winter working and beachcombing? A nursing home?

He had to be talking about two strangers. One was the man outside his office, stooped in his wheelchair, lined up against the wall with a dozen other people in wheelchairs, waiting to be fed. My Limey, for whom privacy had been paramount, who could not bear to have strangers touch him, and who now had to call for an aide to move him an inch or two because the paralysis would not permit him to move his own body. His face was drawn and gray, his clothes hung on his almost six-foot frame, now down to around 115 pounds. He could hold his special spoon in his right hand if someone put it there, and he could manage to get most of his food into his mouth. What he dropped fell into a foolish bib tied around his neck, and was then helped into his mouth by an aide. He drooled because he could not always swallow his saliva. But he could think and he could talk, and at times he talked a lot. Angry talk. "Get me out of this goddamned chair. I want to go back to bed. This chair is torture. I'm sitting on my balls and it hurts. Anyway this food isn't fit to eat, all covered with greasy gravy . . . Why the hell don't they let me die?"

And the doctor was talking about a pale, frightened woman who had fantasized that when her husband was discharged from this rehab center she would take home with her some of her old Limey. She had accepted the fact that he would never walk again—that could be dealt with—but her hope had been that somehow he would be more accepting of his tragedy, that some of his humor, which he had held on to in the beginning, would come back, and that he would not be so totally involved with the torture of his body. She had imagined that he might ask where his wife had been, what she was doing, how her new book was coming along, ask about the children, friends . . . that there would be communication with the outside world that went beyond the unhappy limits of his miserable, spastic limbs.

"What are you going to do?" the doctor repeated, looking at me and also at his watch. He was a busy man.

"I am going to take him home," I said flatly. I looked at him for just a few seconds. I couldn't bear the familiar expression of pity and skepticism.

"We tried our best," he said. "I've never seen our staff work so hard for anyone."

"I know."

I know, I know, I know . . . I could say the words over and over again, but what I didn't know was so overwhelming. "Your husband can live a long time . . ."

Why had those words frightened me? I didn't think I wanted Limey to die. Death was so goddamned final. But what did he have to live for? And what would my life be like?

On a soft, warm day in July, Limey came home. His homecoming was different from what it had been before, and I almost wished for his former hostility. This time he went into a terrible, unrelieved depression. I shared it with him. We didn't talk about it, but now we knew that this was it. Later he sometimes said, "When I get well again," but more often he spoke of wanting to die. I think we both knew that there was going to be no rehabilitation, and my goal now was to maintain the status quo. I was terrified of his getting worse.

What the status quo truly was, was hard to evaluate. It fluctuated. Not his physical handicaps, but his mind, and his mind was what concerned me most, or perhaps I should say his mind and his attitude. We settled into a routine of sorts with the nurse's aide coming in the mornings—a rather tense woman who, because she also had an afternoon job, seemed to worry about getting away on time from the moment she arrived. It got so that she was giving Limey his lunch earlier and earlier to be sure she'd have him finished and ready to go back to bed the minute Millie came in the door and was ready to help her. I found myself getting very annoyed but soon decided it wasn't worth making her more tense than she was. Limey didn't seem to mind getting his lunch at eleven in the morning, so I thought to hell with it. You don't want to lose someone, so you decide what is important and what is not, and although I could not warm up to her, she did her job adequately well.

Actually I looked forward to the Thursday afternoons when Limey and I were alone. It was nice not to have anyone else around, and while I regretted that I could not get him out of bed by myself, he certainly was happy enough to skip the wheelchair. Often I read to him. Limey had always hated being read to. He hadn't liked lectures either; he wanted to see the written or printed words on the paper himself. But now he seemed to enjoy my reading, and I admired the turnabout: he was trying in some way to adapt to a terrible situation. It was the same with the "Talking Records." He still didn't like them, but he did give several of them a try.

I read the beautiful short stories of Isaac Bashevis Singer. Many times I felt sure that Limey had fallen asleep while I was reading, but I did not stop, because, astonishingly, although he did not seem to be listening, later in the evening or the next day he would talk about the story in detail, and even quote whole phrases or sentences to me.

I have made a great point in this book of Limey's lucidity and alertness and his extraordinary memory. Yet the hardest part of his whole illness was, for me, the condition of his mind. According to all the professionals, the doctors and the nurses, Limey was "alert." But their frame of reference seemed to me mechanical; they appeared to me to have a narrow medical standard for the mind rather than a broader, social one. Limey was lucid, he could answer their questions, and he knew who he was and where he was. He was aware. But what had deteriorated so tragically was his ability to absorb any fact (even something so simple as whether he'd had his breakfast or his lunch) and to turn his interest away from himself. Yet it is difficult to say whether his constant verbalization about his body and his repetitiveness were attributable to his mind or his psyche. The fact that he did remember and talk about what I'd read to him and the lucid dictations he put on his tape recorder lead me to believe that the problems of personality and psyche have not been delved into sufficiently by any of the specialists dealing with the effects of stroke.

I once asked Dr. Stern if there was a psychiatrist on their staff. He said no, but that they sometimes called one in from the outside. I suggested that Limey might be helped by one, but he did not encourage it. When Limey was home a psychologist friend offered to spend some time with him, but after two sessions, Limey, as she put it, "fired" her. He did not want to go into any discussions, even though they were on an informal basis. Limey had had some therapy after his first stroke, five years previous, but he had given that up too because he did not find it useful.

I believe that a person's personality has a great deal to do with the handling of a long illness, or perhaps any illness. Limey was not a good candidate for what happened to him. While he was capable of enjoying many things, he had a cynical view of life, and any trouble sent him huddling within himself. Together with his fine mind he also had a certain rigidity in his thinking and in his habits. If he set up a morning routine for himself, he compulsively held to that routine even when he was traveling and it became impractical.

When his tapes were transcribed, it was hard to believe that the same man had dictated them who also screamed at us, "Take me up the ramp" (which meant going back to bed), who was asking to have his eyes wiped dry, who was asking where his hand was, who was begging to die one minute and worrying about his diet the next. Who could also just stare into space as if he weren't thinking at all. But he was. He must have been. He was living within his own thoughts.

Someone once said that when he came to visit Limey, he felt embarrassed. "I spoke to him as if he weren't all there because he only said, 'Move my hand, fix my pillow,' and so forth . . . but I knew his mind was working, although I could not communicate with him on the level of his thoughts." Here are some of them, dictated in August, September and October, after he came home from the rehab center.

It is interesting that on the night that I thought I was going to die any minute and I called Hila out of her sleep, I was not concerned about the problem of dying at all, only that it should be disgraceful if I died without seeing my dear sons and daughters again. That is, my sons and daughters-in-law, of course. I must see them, was what I said. I told Hila, I must see my sons and daughters again, I must see my children. But dying I didn't care about. I would be all right, I would be okay. That was what I expected, anyway.

Another poem—"The Trees Across the Road" is the title.

Across the road the trees are taller and more leafy than those
     in the dog run or closer
Nor do they wither quite so early
They're green now that the others are all brown, or red or
     faded
The trees across the road are straight and tall and leafy
Across the road they're thick like my grandfather's beard
Everything is always better somewhere else
Like across the road, for example

How I must look to Hila when she takes care of me:

I must be an awfully strange and not at all admirable character to her because she would be proud of me if I were stoic and I guess I'm anything but that. I scream when she has to clean me or when she does anything that hurts me in the course of taking care of me, which often happens unavoidably. I don't respond too well either when she asks me to do certain things that would be helpful to her in the process of helping me. This is perhaps how I look to Hila. I must look like an awfully stupid fart; a very cowardly fart, I must be in her sight and hearing. I guess I'm just not fit to be the husband of anyone with a stoic ideal. I guess that's my problem. Of course the whole thing is my problem not Hila's, because I'm the one who's at fault.

There is a bowl of crab apples sitting on the sofa here. The sofa has a blue and white pattern slipcover and the bowl is blue and white, sort of a Chinese blue. The crab apples are crab-apple color. They're so beautiful in that bowl. I just moved them from one bowl to another for exercise of my fingers and it's difficult to move even the crab apple with the back of one's hand. I found that out.

I must appear really like a horse's ass a lot of the time. I'm very garrulous, as anybody knows. And I guess I keep talking, talking, talking, talking, and maybe what I say makes sense and maybe it doesn't, but most likely not because why should that make sense. And I don't other ways, in any case.

And the other people who work with me also say I'm very garrulous. And they can't stand my talking all the time while they're working with me.

That last poem of mine about the autumn rains makes me think about the delicacy of nature's balance. Nature is not a Rockefeller type sitting in a Wall Street office making checks and balances and figuring out his dimes and nickels. Nature doesn't have to balance even though it apparently does—that is, I think, an illusion. I think the balance part of it is a human artifact, a convenient way of referring to certain phenomena.

Up above there, nature is not some cheap Rockefeller banker type. Nature is everything in the world, so what the hell does it need this penny-pinching shit for.

To explain some otherwise inexplicable phenomena.

Nature does not have to make a red tree for every green tree or anything like that. Nature is all and its own mistress, and entirely her own mistress. It is not even correct to say that what goes up must come down, although it could be said perhaps that what goes up may come down. It would probably be correct to say that what goes up may come down, or what may go up may come down. So let's not have any of these easy "balances" again, not even in a poem where it is most likely to be misunderstood and taken too seriously. Balance is an artificial thing which I can put in a poem but don't blame nature for it or its presence there.

Balance is a formal thing. You may notice that the closer to the primitive the less formal its design. Look at your children's drawings; that is, the drawings made by your children before any teacher has had the opportunity to ruin their approach. They have no form, certainly no formality. I had some made by a niece and nephew of eight years old. They were made perhaps fifty years ago, I wish I had them now, they were so beautiful. Let's say, very attractive, and showed more sense than many drawings by older people.

How could I not have remembered that Limey expressed his feelings best with words on paper—and even though these pieces were dictated, are repetitive and far from Limey's normal sparse, polished writing, he thought of them as written. He could not read them. He could not read at all. His recent verbosity—inconsequential chatter —had misled me and kept luring me into thinking that he was paying no attention. There was often a span of weeks before I got a tape transcribed, and each time I read a new one, my hopes rose. When he was alone in his room and was silent, when he could not sleep at night, that man was thinking, he was still making notes for his book. Behind the childish chatter and within that broken body Limey was still so aware. He was alive.

We can go on this way for years, I thought, and yet I felt peculiarly suspended in time. And in place too. While my communication, my feeling of intimacy and closeness to Limey, was cut down to those times when we were alone—not too frequent and a good deal of that time he was asleep—I felt more closely bound up with him than I guess I ever had been. I no longer had the release of getting angry. You could not be angry with Limey now—he was too docile, too acquiescent, he had lost his anger, and he seemed to know that with his work he was waging a losing battle against time. I knew there was nothing more to do now than to try to keep him as comfortable as possible, and I tried to do that. I still insisted on the wheelchair, but with less rigidity, and when he was tired we let him rest in bed.

It was when I was away from home, out with friends, that I felt an unreality, felt like a displaced person. Going to a dinner party with Limey and going alone were two totally different experiences. Limey's provocative presence was conspicuously absent. I had to face the reality that my life was going to be led on two levels: my demanding but limited life with Limey, and a life I would have to make for myself alone. It was a learning process. Learning to walk in the woods alone with Jo, learning to enjoy a sunset that Limey could not see, to enjoy a movie, an evening out with friends, to watch a show on television while Limey was asleep. I shared whatever I could with Limey—bringing home something from the woods for him, reading an amusing or interesting tidbit from the newspaper—and I depended heavily on our friends, whose warmth I cannot exaggerate. They came to see him although I know it was painful for many of them, and I hardly went to a dinner party without my hostess plying me with portions to take home for Limey.

Occasionally I was able to lull myself into a deluded,

nostalgic few hours. When we were home alone, even though Limey couldn't see me very well, I'd get out of my jeans, wash my face, put on a long caftan, and settle down with a drink and my dinner and a TV program or a book, and for a while I'd think, oh well, it's not all that different—he's just in the next room having a nap, as he used to do sometimes, and here I am.

When people asked me, "How are you? How are you managing?" I didn't know how to answer. Simple answers would have been easy, but they were never right. If I said, "Fine," they looked at me as if I were some kind of idiotic, self-sacrificing heroine, which God knows I wasn't, nor did I want to be. On the other hand, when I said, "It's rough," which was much closer to the truth, they felt sorry for me, which I didn't want either, nor did I want to be a chronic complainer. How did I manage? The answer is complicated, perhaps both as complicated and as simple as any part of life is. I had good days and bad days, and often I felt like the person who takes on one big debt to pay off all his little debts. I had one central problem, or anxiety if you will, and as a result so many of the lesser aggravations I had found disturbing in the past became unimportant. It's all relative. Minor crises like the washing machine breaking down (we had Limey's sheets and towels and so forth to do every day), or an electric storm cutting off our power when Limey's electrically operated hospital bed was in a sitting position and we couldn't get the hand crank to put it down, became funny. You learned to grab on to whatever came your way to relieve the grimness, to bring laughter into the house. I got to like having Millie and the nurse's aide around—they were able to laugh with me at the way Limey ordered his harem around and were good-natured about Limey's four-letter words and his idiosyncrasies. Often he made a big thing out of what shirt he wanted to wear, and he was specific about what he wanted. At night when we were getting him undressed and into pajamas, he went through a regular patter of telling us that he didn't want to wear pajamas, that they bound him, and that we couldn't possibly get anything on him. In fact, all of Limey's clothing was very loose, but he complained a great deal of feeling bound by them; actually it was his paralysis that made him feel constricted. Dressing him and undressing him was not easy; getting his unbending arms through sleeves was a painstaking job, and you had to give up worrying about ripping the armholes of even his favorite shirts. But it was good for his morale and for mine to see him dressed, so we stuck to it.

Fortunately I have a capacity for enjoying myself, and I am interested in everything that goes on around me: in people, politics, books, movies, the weather, food, money, walking, talking . . . I still had all these things to keep me going, as well as my writing. But it was something I had to work at. I was extremely restless. My attention span at the typewriter was considerably shorter than normal. I had to, I wanted to, get up every now and then and go in to see what was going on with Limey; I went out for shorter but more frequent walks; I spoke with friends on the phone more often—I couldn't sit still for long. When I went away from home, after a couple of hours I needed to get right back.

But I was learning to accept the reality of what was, and to know that what I could not change, I could not change. When Limey was brighter than usual I was grateful. When I went to bed at night I was glad if he gave me a solid kiss and seemed reasonably comfortable, although the question often haunted me, would I be relieved if he died quietly in his sleep? I always put that question aside: maybe five years from now I could be, but not now, not yet . . . not while I could still cope and Limey's mind was as good as it was.

I don't think anyone realized, and I didn't myself, how much strength, such as I had, I got from Limey. As Dr. Stern had said, no one knew the nightmare he was living in, but in spite of all his protestations, his saying he wanted to die, he was summoning up tremendous energy to live. Everything was such a monumental effort for him: to eat, to be dressed, to be moved, to sit in the wheelchair, to work at his tape recorder, to try, with such frustration, to punch wrong letters on his typewriter, to want visitors and yet be exhausted after a brief time. When I was having trouble hammering a nail in straight—something Limey used to do so easily—I could imagine one-millionth of the frustration, the terrible helplessness, he was suffering, and my heart went out to him, but with an admiration that was a terrific boost for me. When I found myself slipping into self-pity (which I certainly was not free of), I had to think: I can walk, run, skip, I can go out of the house, I can enjoy food, a drink, I can get in the car and drive, I can do anything, and everything that he cannot. I must never lose sight of that. And yet, when he woke me up in the middle of the night to tell me that he felt abandoned, my emotions were familiarly ambivalent: oh God, why did he have to wake me up to tell me this now, and how sad that he did.

One evening I attempted a dinner party. A few close friends were invited, including Limey's doctor and his wife—having them there gave me a much needed feeling of security. We let Limey rest in bed all afternoon and only got him up and wheeled him into the living room when the guests arrived. In spite of his gauntness he looked handsome in his favorite Mexican shirt, and although he had had his supper earlier, at his usual time, he sipped at a drink and ate some of the hors d'oeuvres. That evening is printed indelibly on my mind. God knows, Limey and I had given hundreds of dinner parties in the past, but the pleasure of having him there then, of having a time together, with friends, that to some degree approximated a normal life, was tremendous. It was a good party.

I do believe that, after all, the secret of managing is to try to keep one's life with an invalid as close as possible to the ordinary, everyday way one lived before. I have thought about the people who, when faced with a terminal illness, have wanted to go around the world, or spend their time in some exotic or romantic pursuit, and I cannot help believing that the pleasure they find must be hard to come by. To me, any move that dramatizes an illness, or any tragedy for that matter, can only emphasize the pain. To keep an even keel, I found for myself and for Limey, we had to look to the same distractions and the same pleasures that we knew and that had worked in the past to keep us from abandoning ourselves to disaster.

We had structured our lives and our interests in a certain way, and I found that following the same pattern was the most comforting and secure. I was not interested in meeting new people; I wanted only my old, familiar, time-tested friends. I wanted our daily routine to be as close as possible to what it had been before—I did not long for a change. Some friends asked, "Can't you arrange to get away for a few days?" Maybe I could have, but I didn't want to. I wanted to stick close to home. I counted on the small things that had made up our life together before to stand by us now and lighten the weight of our tragedy. And most of all, for my sake as much as Limey's, I wanted to keep alive, without a break on my part, whatever threads of communication we had going for us, and that depended on small, daily happenings in the household, discussing the preparation of a special dish with Limey, watching a TV show with him, reading mail to him. In essence we were hanging on to a way of life that was familiar and tried, and the threat we feared was any new change.

A change came. I think it was foreshadowed one Sunday morning in early October. A Sunday, of course, when the Sunday nurse had called to say that she could not come in. I went into Limey's room in the morning and found that the urinal bag was empty and that his genitals were red and considerably swollen. Immediately I called our family doctor, but, as might be expected, he was out of town. I called the doctor who was covering for him and he told me on the phone to put cold compresses on my husband and said that he would check with me later in the afternoon. I was not impressed with this advice. I was really scared. Limey did not complain of pain, but he did not want to eat. What to do?

In desperation I called a friend who lived in town, a doctor who was not in private practice but who was connected with a hospital in a neighboring city. When I told him the situation, he promptly said, "He has to be catheterized." That was what I had thought.

Thank God for people like Dr. Patten. He left his family that Sunday, drove some thirty miles to get the equipment he needed, and in a remarkably short time was at Limey's bedside catheterizing him. He also discovered that Limey was impacted and proceeded to take care of that. (It was only then that I learned that runny, watery feces can indicate an impaction.) Limey was exhausted when the doctor finished and he fell into a deep sleep. My instructions were to feed him lightly (which we did pretty much anyway), and to keep track of his liquid intake and output.

Dr. Patten left a very grateful and relieved woman behind him. I also became abruptly aware of a great naïveté on my part. Taking care of Limey had meant to me working with and around the results of his stroke. I had never thought about other internal complications. I don't know why I had been so dumb. Of course, the visiting nurse had been explicit about keeping his bowels open and we had given him medication to that end, but I had never thought about it as a serious problem. In any event, my sense of relief was short-lived. By four or five in the afternoon Limey was still sleeping, and when I tried to wake him up to give him something to drink, and eat too, I hoped, I could not rouse him. I patted his cheeks, I shook him gently, I did everything I could, but he would not wake up.

Coma was the first thing that came into my mind. In panic I called Dr. Patten again and he came right over. After examining him, he said, "His life signs are all okay. He's just very tired. He'll be all right."

Limey was all right, but the episode marked a setback for him. For a few days his speech was affected, he could not feed himself—could not get the spoon to his mouth at all—and he was very drowsy. Dr. Patten told me that any upset could affect a stroke patient that way, but that the retrogression would be temporary. It was an agonizing few days. I had to trust Dr. Patten, but I couldn't be sure. He was marvelous. For the next couple of days he came to see Limey in the morning before he went to the hospital and again late in the evening when he came back.

I was dying to ask him if he would take Limey on as a patient, since he was so dedicated and lived nearby. While

I loved our family doctor I knew he was extremely busy and made as few house calls as possible. So when Limey improved, as the doctor had said he would, I did ask him. Dr. Patten said that he would work with another doctor, and we went through a list of names that he suggested. On his recommendation we agreed on one, and Dr. Patten called him from my house and explained the situation. "I will do the house calls," he said, "but most of what is needed you can do on the phone, once you have seen the patient."

The man at the other end of the phone apparently needed some coaxing about caring for a paraplegic at home. Dr. Patten said, "There's a very good setup here. He is very well taken care of and there is full-time help. It's all right."

So there was agreement and the next step was to make an appointment for Dr. Harris to come to see Limey. In the meantime I felt obligated to call our family doctor, to bring him up to date on what had happened and to tell him of the new plan. He knew Dr. Patten and agreed that it made sense for us, and while I felt regret in giving up our family doctor at this point—Limey was very fond of him, he had taken care of us and our sons for years, and I had affection and respect for him—I felt that I needed someone who would be available in an emergency. Indeed I felt lucky that Dr. Patten, a man with highly qualified background and training, with a personal dedication, and so conveniently nearby, had arranged this team of two to take on Limey. When it was all done I felt secure, but thinking about it and feeling my way through that mysterious world of medical diplomacy was nerve-wracking.

I liked Dr. Harris. After he examined Limey, he came into the kitchen and sat down and talked to me. "I am concerned about you," he said. "Your welfare is as important as your husband's. How are you getting along?"

"I'm hanging on."

"What can I do to help you?" He was very direct. I had to think a few minutes before answering.

"Perhaps if I ever got around to taking a vacation, maybe in the spring, you could help me find someone to stay here. I'd keep the help I have, but I'd want someone very responsible in the house."

"That's not easy," he said. "Even if you're willing to spend a lot of money. But you can put your husband into a nursing home for a month or so. It would be better than trying to get someone to stay here. We do that all the time. He would know it was temporary."

It was a new idea that had never occurred to me. Much as I wanted to stick close to home there were times when I felt trapped by the situation. The thought that a vacation might be possible at some point was comforting, whether I ever took advantage of it or not. To know that a door had been opened would relieve the trapped feeling when it hit me. I felt that Dr. Harris was really concerned about me. He also said something before he left that I had reason to remember later. "I want to do enough for your husband," he said, "but not too much." I made no comment, but I sensed that he was telling me that he would not do anything extraordinary to keep my husband alive.

So the days and a couple of weeks went by, blessedly uneventful. Things were going smoothly enough for me to plan to take my son and daughter-in-law and two of my grandchildren to a theater in Hartford where a friend was in a play. When I left home in the middle of the afternoon all was in order. I expected to get back late, and since Millie did not want to stay, a practical nurse was to come in at five o'clock to help Millie get Limey out of the wheelchair and into bed, and to stay the night. It was raining quite heavily when I left, but I was thankful it was rain and not snow and gave it little further thought. I was looking forward to the evening and felt lucky that I had found someone to come in so that I could have a night out with my kids.

When I arrived at my son's house I called home to make sure everything was all right. Millie said, "The Fire Department called to see if we were okay."

"Why? What happened? Why should they call?"

"I guess because of the rain," she said vaguely. "I told them we were fine."

"What about the nurse? She should be there by now."

"I guess she'll be along soon. We're okay, don't worry," said Millie.

It sounded very peculiar to me, and a little while later I called again. "Did Mrs. Frank arrive?" I was surprised that Millie was still there.

"The Fire Department told me they would try to bring her in, but they didn't."

"What in God's name are you talking about? Millie, what has happened?" I had a very uneasy feeling that Millie had found our liquor closet.

"I think the road's been washed out. But we're all right, we're fine."

"Good God, from the rain! You'll have to stay, Millie."

She giggled. "If she can't come in, I can't get out." At least she was making sense.

"How is Mr. Colman?"

"He's fine. He said he wished he could see what was going on. Go on and have a good time. Don't worry about us."

Don't worry . . . famous words. My kids, however, reassured me. "There's nothing you can do now, so relax. Millie knows how to take care of him, and you couldn't get home anyway if the road is washed out."

At this point the radio was saying that there had been some flooded areas but that the rain was going to stop during the night. It was hard to think of our gentle stream washing out the road, but I did have the memory of the 1955 flood, and I knew what our brook could do, although even at that time our house had not been touched. There was nothing that I could do. Later I found that neighbors who knew that I was away for the evening had called our house and couldn't believe Millie's nonchalance. I was pretty sure she had fortified herself with a liquid protection. I never asked her, but I could hardly blame her.

It was still raining when we came out of the theater. My son wanted me to stay the night with them, but I wanted to get as close to home as possible. Fortunately the son of my actress friend had flown up from Washington to see his mother in the play, and he suggested that he drive me back to their house, which was not far from ours. The rain had not let up and it was a harrowing drive. What ordinarily took around an hour took us more than three—we went through flooded roads and pelting rain. I was still awake around four in the morning, when I had a horrible thought. In my agitated state I had completely forgotten to ask Millie how she got Limey back to bed. He had been in the wheelchair when I'd left. She had never done it alone, and I had the frightening thought of Limey sitting up in the wheelchair all night. I lay in bed trying to keep myself from going to the phone. There was no point in calling her then. If he was in the wheelchair there was nothing I could do about it on the phone, and if he was safely in bed, and they were both asleep, there was no sense in awakening them.

I did not sleep much that night. I waited until seven o'clock in the morning to get up, get dressed, and leave. By that time it had stopped raining. I had no trouble driving to the start of our country road, but there I was stopped by signs that said ROAD CLOSED. I parked the car, and, in my long skirt and high heels, proceeded to walk toward our house. I came to what looked like a bombed-out area. Where the brook crossed under the road above our house, there was no road. The town crew was working in a mass of rubble and rocks some eight feet deep. They greeted me cheerfully, assured me that things were all right down at my house, and helped me climb down, stepping from rock to rock, and then climb up the six or eight feet on the other side onto the road. The same condition existed below our house where the stream crossed again. Our house was on an isolated island.

I picked up my skirt and ran the rest of the way home. I ran right into Limey's room, and there he was, sitting up in bed as if nothing had happened at all. "You got him into bed, Millie." I hugged her. "You are wonderful. How did you do it?"

She grinned. "I said to Mr. Colman, 'It's just you and me, and I'm going to get you into bed.' If you have to do it, you do it." Then she added slyly, "I'd just as soon you didn't know I could do it alone."

I laughed with her. "I'm glad I do know. But don't worry, I won't take advantage of you."

It wasn't until late that evening that the road was temporarily fixed and Millie could get her car out and I could get mine in. But I couldn't have cared less. God knows, a flood was the last thing I had on my list of worries, but if we came through that intact we were in pretty good shape. In a way, the flood gave me a lighthearted feeling, a sense of security that I could count on Millie in a crisis.

My euphoria was short-lived. In the ensuing weeks Millie became more and more peculiar. It is possible that the night of the flood could have started her on a bout with liquor. The day that she came in forgetting how to make Jell-O, a dessert she had been making several times a week for Limey for several months, I realized that something had to be done. But what? I was in a quandary. She did have good qualities, but her vagueness and confusion often mixed her up about when she was supposed to come in, and her outright forgetfulness was getting to be too much.

I had to be on hand all the time to see that he got his exercises, that his meals were prepared and given to him, that his clothes and linens got washed—I was paying her well and cheerfulness alone wasn't enough. I was getting annoyed with her intense ritual of watching the afternoon soap operas while Limey needed attention. I discussed the problem with the visiting nurse, who was as aware of the situation as I, and she suggested that I call the office that sent out the nurse's aides and homemakers, the Family and Children's Aid, a volunteer agency supported by the United Fund and private donations. This is a fine organization that provides able personnel either as homemakers, people to cook and help in homes where there are disabled elderly or children who need care and the families cannot afford to pay for help, or, as in our case, nurse's aides for the sick, who come under the Medicare program. They also provide family counseling. I spoke to an intelligent, understanding woman on the phone who said that she would get back to me. I couldn't believe it when she called back in a few hours and told me that she could have a nurse's aide for me for the whole day, from 8 A.M. until 6 P.M. "We have some money," she said, "and I have someone available."

"You mean for the whole day, free?" It didn't seem possible.

"That's right. She can start on Monday if you want."

I certainly did want. It was hard to believe, and for a

brief while I was furious that no one had told me about this before. I started to count up in my head all the money I would have saved, plus having someone with some training, and then sternly told myself to forget it. It was only money, and besides there must be a hitch to it, it couldn't last, and I talked myself into thinking it was just as well I had Millie as a backup.

I later learned that the Family and Children's Aid was able to provide a full-time person for me at that time because of a special grant received from the Federal Commission on Aging. It was a matching-funds arrangement, with the federal government giving 75 percent and the agency raising the other 25 percent. Since then it has been changed to 50 percent from each, and in another year the government grant will be cut even more. It is a pity, and it seems to me totally wrong and shortsighted to cut back on this kind of program, which provides for home care that is more economical, and in most cases far more satisfactory, than institutional care.

The next step, which I dreaded, was to tell Millie. I did not want to sever my relations with her, so the proper diplomacy was essential. Since this was Friday and the nurse's aide was to start on Monday, there was no time for any notice. However, I decided to give Millie a week's salary, and to tell her only the truth: that the nurse's aide would be free, and since Millie knew about money and was aware that I did not have much of it, she would understand that part of it. Also that I did not know how long it would last, similarly true, and that she should check with me before she took another job. I doubted

very much, and not without justification, that Millie was
going to look for another job.

Still, I put off telling her until Saturday. Saturday
turned out to be one of those golden fall days we get in
Connecticut—it was early November now—and I had an
irresistible urge to get out. It so happened that our
younger son was down from Cambridge visiting his older
brother, and I decided I would drive up and spend a few
hours with them. Limey's brother Morris had been in the
habit of coming to see him every Saturday, and after making sure that he was going to be at our house (I didn't feel
easy about leaving Millie alone for several hours), I left,
after Limey's lunch, while he was in his bed resting. He
hadn't been hungry for lunch—had had some trouble
chewing and swallowing a hamburger, but this had happened before on occasion, so it didn't alarm me. We gave
him a couple of soft-boiled eggs instead, and he ate those
all right. "If he feels like getting up when Morris comes,"
I told Millie, "all right, but don't push him. Let him rest
in bed if he wants to." Limey always enjoyed his brother's
visits. They spoke a good deal about their family and their
childhood as well as the times when they'd been together
as young men. They had a great affection for each other,
and I knew I wouldn't be missed. I planned to get home
before Millie was to leave at six.

The drive to my son's house is a pleasant one, and I was
in good spirits. The new arrangement to begin on Monday was a big lift, and I was already figuring that with
the money I would save perhaps I could really put Limey
in a nursing home for a month and take a vacation in the

spring. When I arrived I was glad to find that everyone, including all the children, wanted to be outdoors as much as I, and we embarked on a long hike through a wooded and quite wild state park near my son's house. It was a beautiful walk that took around three hours. Of course, I wished Limey could have been with us—it was the kind of expedition he loved to go on with the family—but I did feel that things at home were working out better than I had expected.

When we got back to Jonny's house, I was going to take off for home but as a routine matter called there first to check.

"Mr. Colman's in the hospital," Millie's voice said over the phone. "He's in the —— hospital," she said, naming a hospital in a city near our home, the one with which Dr. Patten and Dr. Harris were affiliated. "His brother took him there."

"What happened?" I was surprised that I was able to speak.

"He wouldn't wake up. Morris called the doctor and the doctor said to take him in the ambulance to the emergency. Morris tried to call you."

"We were out walking," I said stupidly.

"Should I wait here?" Millie asked.

"I don't care . . . No, you can go home. If I need you I'll call you. I'll go straight to the hospital. Millie, did he wake up when they took him?"

"I don't know," she said.

I had to sit quietly by myself for a few minutes before I went outside to tell the boys. Thank God Morris was there, I thought, and I reminded myself that it wasn't pure luck. I wouldn't have gone off, even for these few hours, without knowing he would be there. I also clung to the fact that once before I couldn't awaken Limey but he had been all right.

Tacitly we all underplayed the turn of events. "No, don't come with me," I said to my sons. "I'll be all right. I'll call you from the hospital."

"Call now and see if you can talk to Morris," Jonny said.

I got Morris on the phone and he told me the same thing Millie had. "He's upstairs now, getting X-rays," Morris added. "So I don't know anything more yet."

"I'll get there as soon as I can."

"Drive carefully," Morris said.

I drove fast, and I hadn't been putting up a false bravado when I'd told the boys not to come with me. I was trying desperately to play it down and didn't want anything that suggested a terrible crisis. Morris had probably just gotten alarmed . . . I tried to think about the beautiful walk we had had, how lively and delightful the grandchildren had been, how lucky I was to have such a family—they were my main source of pleasure now— but the thought kept rearing its ugly head, had Limey been dying while we were out walking?

The emergency room was busy and crowded and nowhere could I find Morris. Then I spied Limey lying flat on a table, alone, covered with a sheet. I ran over to him. He opened his eyes, but he didn't say anything. I bent down and kissed him, and murmured things like "I love you . . . You're going to be all right . . . Can you hear me? Can you speak to me? I love you . . ."

His eyes followed me, and once he spoke in a hoarse whisper, "Hi-la, Hi-la, Hi-la . . ." And that was all.

At the nurse's desk, no one could tell me anything. "Miss Holmes knows, she's busy, she'll be with you soon," was all the information I could get. I scanned the waiting room again in search of Morris, but he was nowhere to be found.

I was ready to stand in the middle of the floor and scream, "Someone tell me what is going on with my husband," when finally Miss Holmes turned up. "You'll have to talk to the doctor who admitted him," she told me. "I think he's up in the X-ray room; you can call him." She led me to a phone and I dialed the extension number she gave me.

I got the doctor on the phone, and the first thing he did was to yell at me. "What kind of a shitty family have you got? I'm glad at least someone is interested in this man . . ."

"What in hell are you talking about?" I yelled back at him. "This man is my husband—he came in in an emergency and he is probably the best-cared-for man in the state of Connecticut. I wasn't home when he was brought here in an ambulance."

"I had him up for X-rays and when I brought him down there was no one there. I used to be at Bellevue in New York and I saw this happen too many times, I've seen patients dumped . . ."

"He wasn't dumped. Now tell me what you've found."

"I don't know yet. But I'm admitting him to the hospital. There'll be a bed for him on the fourth floor, Room 406. Will you go up with him?"

"Of course I will."

The nurse in charge was sympathetic. "He's odd," she said. "Don't pay any attention. He even put on his chart that Mr. Colman was abandoned. I'm going to take it right off."

"I really don't care what's on his chart," I said, furious.

I stood by Limey until they were ready to take him upstairs. He opened his eyes a few times, and I know he knew I was with him, but he didn't speak. We were still downstairs when suddenly a dear friend, Dallas, appeared. Dallas was a young woman who had lived with us for a while when the boys were small, and we thought of her as part of the family. I was completely astonished to see her.

She explained that she had stopped by our house to visit Limey, and when Morris took him in the ambulance to the hospital, she had followed in her car. While Limey was in the X-ray room, Morris had tried to call his wife, whom he was supposed to meet someplace, but couldn't reach her. Also it was getting late, and Morris, a man in his middle seventies, didn't favor driving in the dark. So Dallas had taken him back to our house to get his car so that he could go on home. Of course, no one had been there when Limey came down from the X-ray room. So much for the irate doctor, although by that time I had gotten around to thinking that it was rather nice that he had been so concerned.

I was very glad to have Dallas with me. She gave me tremendous support, and I think that night we formed a bond that will never be broken. We stayed with Limey until he was safely settled in a bed in a room that had one other, unoccupied bed in it. I sat with him awhile, and finally we left.

It was close to eleven o'clock by that time. Dallas offered to come home with me, but I assured her that I would be all right. When I got home I reported to the boys and to Morris, but there was very little to tell them. I really didn't know what had happened. All I knew was that Morris had not been able to awaken Limey, that he had called Dr. Patten, who was out of town, and that an associate of his had told Morris to bring Limey right down to the emergency room.

The next morning my dear friend Ses was at my house early; we got hold of Dr. Wolf, the neurologist, who was at his country weekend place nearby, and he and his wife accompanied us to the hospital. Fortunately Dr. Harris was there at the same time. Limey was motionless, being fed intravenously once again, and he was not speaking. But I was sure his eyes acknowledged me.

There was no certain diagnosis and no prognosis. "It's too soon to tell anything," the doctors told me. "It looks very much as if he's had another stroke, but it's hard to tell. We'll just have to wait and see."

Wait and see . . . wait and see . . . Now there was no ducking it. Was I waiting for him to die? I could not answer that question. I was just waiting, in suspension. When I was home, each time the phone rang I was afraid to answer. I went to the hospital every day. Often Ses accompanied me. The boys came, my daughters-in-law came. Dallas came often and so did her brother, whom Limey had known and loved since he was a baby. It became clear that Limey had had another stroke. His speech was lost, and now he was motionless. He did not move even his right arm or leg. I was glad to have those close to us there, but I also liked to sit with him alone. We were all sure that he knew when we were there, and when I was alone with him I felt a certain kind of peacefulness. Limey had never been afraid of death, and I didn't think he was afraid now.

I cannot bear people who say of someone who is unable to communicate, "He doesn't understand anyway." How do they know? How does anyone know? I was grateful to the nurses for their sensitivity and tenderness, not only toward Limey but also toward my feelings: Limey was still a person, a man to be treated with dignity, and that meant a lot to me. Patiently they explained to him everything that they had to do, assuming that he understood. They wheeled him out into the solarium, where he stared out the window. Sometimes I wasn't sure that he did know. "Can you blink your eyes and let me know that you can hear me?" I asked him, but his eyes did not move.

Once, when Dallas was standing beside me, in that same hoarse, whispering voice I had heard the first night, he said my name, "Hi-la, Hi-la, Hi-la." I would have thought I'd imagined it if Dallas had not heard it too.

Limey had been in that same condition for almost three weeks when Dr. Harris said to me, "I'm going to take him off the IV" (the intravenous). I had told him, and the boys had told him, that we did not want Limey kept artificially alive. Jimmy had shown him a letter Limey had written expressing that as his own wish.

"What are you going to do?"

"We'll try to feed him orally. He's getting practically nothing in the IV anyway."

"I don't think he can swallow. Isn't that an awful way to die? To starve to death?"

"He feels very little, if at all. Will you trust me?" Dr. Harris asked.

I hesitated barely a few seconds. "Yes, I trust you," I said. And I knew that Limey would have been grateful.

We had that conversation the day before Thanksgiving. I alerted the boys to what was going on, but thank God they, like me, had no stomach for a death watch. Whatever our private thoughts, no one voiced aloud a desire to sit around waiting for Limey to die. We went about our daily lives as we had for the past many months. None of us wanted to participate in one of those ghastly huddles to plan our moves: Should the boys wait around or go home? Should I sit at the hospital all day? There is no timetable for death. Each to his own way, and time and place, of meeting it, and as Dr. Toby Wolf once said, "No one dies at the convenience of the relatives." Limey was in my thoughts every minute of the day, but I felt that I would be betraying his own dignity if I sat on edge waiting for him to leave me. When he was ready, he would go.

Jimmy and his family came down from Cambridge for Thanksgiving as we had planned. We spent part of the day at the hospital with Limey but declined the hospital's offer to have our Thanksgiving dinner there. We had a quiet and excellent goose dinner with close friends near home. Jonny and Wanda had dinner with Wanda's family and came down on Friday to see Limey and us. They all went home on Friday evening. They had all been very dear. I felt their warmth even after they were gone, and I did not mind being alone.

On Saturday I had arranged to meet Morris at the hospital for lunch. We wouldn't be allowed to go upstairs until two o'clock. I got there at about twelve-thirty, and as I sat waiting in the lounge the thought crossed my mind that Limey could be dying upstairs while I was sitting there. I was about to go up in the hope that no one would stop me, but then Morris arrived and I said nothing. We went to a nearby Italian restaurant. I don't remember what we talked about, but since we had close to an hour and a half, we ate leisurely and drank some wine.

We got back to the hospital a few minutes before two, and as usual stopped at the desk to get our passes. Only two visitors were allowed to go up at a time.

The woman at the desk said, "Oh, you're going to Mr. Colman. I have to call upstairs first."

I knew instantly that this was it. I grabbed Morris' hand and said, "Something has happened. I know that something has happened." Morris held my hand tightly in his own.

"Go to the nurses' desk, not to the room," the woman said. We did not wait for the elevator but went up the flight of stairs to his floor. We walked rapidly down the corridor and the head nurse came to meet us. I knew by her face what she had to tell me. "My husband died."

The nurse nodded her head. "Yes. Come into the solarium." Morris had his arms around me, and my tears flowed. I was surprised and grateful that I could cry so easily, but then I had been doing that for weeks. Foolishly I kept saying, "I'm sorry . . . I shouldn't be crying, I knew it had to happen . . ." The three of us sat there, with Morris' arms around me. After a while I asked the nurse, "Was he alone?"

"No, he wasn't alone. We were with him."

"Thank you for that. When?"

"About an hour, or an hour and a half ago."

"Then I was sitting downstairs . . ." If only I had followed my instincts and gone up.

"Do you want to see him?" she asked.

I nodded my head. The curtain was drawn around his bed, and there he was, propped up in bed as he had been before, his head to one side, looking like a wounded bird. I kissed his warm forehead and stood with him alone after Morris and the nurse had left me. I was no longer crying, and I knew that his face as I saw it then, no different from what it had been the day before, would be with me for the rest of my life. I did not say goodbye.

Morris took me home and soon our sons and their wives were with me, and after a while friends and country neighbors filled our house with their warmth and affection and gifts of food and drink.

It was all what I believe is called exceedingly "civilized." The tears were quiet. No one sobbed hysterically. But at one time, in that cold, moonlit evening, I went up to our woods alone where no one could hear me and yelled as loud as I could, "Limey, Limey, Limey." I guess that was my farewell.

Epilogue

Limey had always said that he wanted a merry party when he died and I think we gave him what he wanted. We did not give it any name, neither reception nor memorial, we simply asked everyone to come to express their feelings for Limey because we had had no funeral service. For myself it seemed a cross between a Quaker meeting and an Irish wake.

It was in our house on a Sunday in December, a few weeks after Limey died. We had very rarely given big parties, and now I felt totally insane ordering large quantities of liquor and discussing with the man who ran a local catering service the kind of food I wanted. Everything had to be as Limey would have liked.

Our sons and daughters-in-law and all the grandchildren were there early that Sunday morning (some had come the day before) and I woke up feeling I had gone out of my mind. Why had I ever let myself in for this? The boys had felt that we all needed something to mark Limey's leaving us, and I had agreed. But that morning, when the house had been arranged for a party, a bar set up, a large table spread with beautiful food (Limey had always insisted that the look of food was as important as the taste), I wanted to run and hide. To have something so closely resembling a party seemed dreadful. I was in no mood for a party. Also I was sure that no one would come, and I was almost wishing that they wouldn't. But they did. Some fifty or sixty people came, from New York, from the area, some old friends I hadn't seen for a few years.

It was like a party. People ate and drank, the grandchildren ran around, it was very strange. I felt in a daze. Then something extraordinary and wonderful happened. Limey's brother Morris stood up and, leaning against a chair, started to talk informally about Limey. Everyone gathered around, on the floor, on chairs, leaning against tables, and listened. He spoke of their childhood together, their years in Switzerland, he related some amusing and poignant anecdotes of Limey's childhood—nothing was rehearsed, and he was not giving us any eulogies. He just talked about Limey with affection and told many people who were there things they had not known.

When Morris stopped talking, a neighbor, sitting on the floor, picked up and told about how she had first met Limey and her discussion with him about cucumbers. Then someone else spoke of going out to look for morels with Limey, and it went on, with many friends pleasantly reminiscing. Limey's old boss at the pharmaceutical house spoke of how Limey's need for perfection used to drive the typists crazy, but also how they loved him just the same. One friend, Saul, had us all in laughter when he told about a conversation Limey had had with a writer, Louise, about the subjunctive mood. When Louise had died suddenly, Limey had grieved because he loved her but also because he could never finish their discussion of the use of the subjunctive mood. "Limey," he said, "was the protector of language, all language: English, French, Hindi, Chinese, any language. And what's more, he made you feel guilty as hell if you did not do the same. God help you if you abused the English language in his presence."

The day turned out to be the way Limey would have wanted. It was the right farewell for him.

Except that I did not and do not want to say farewell. I want to talk about Limey, I want to think about him, I want to hold on to him. "How could you write this book?" I have been asked. "Isn't it too painful?" Yet I could not help but write this book, I *had* to write it. Because I am a writer by trade, I guess it had to be my way of giving myself something tangible to turn to in the future, besides all the many hours I had alone while writing it, with a reason to sit and think about Limey. It was a good thing to do.

Time heals all wounds, they say, and while I am not one to sit and nurse wounds, I do not want the impact of Limey's life on mine to fade. I enjoy life, and I hope I always will. Martha, a friend who has known me for many years, said, "Hila will stop enjoying herself when the undertaker comes to take her away." I hope she is proven right.

But it is with the quality of that enjoyment that I am more concerned now, and it was Limey, including the painful last year of his illness, who caused me to shift my standards. I am by nature an accepting person, which in a world of multiple choices is not always a good thing to be. There are too many people, too many books, too many movies, too many opportunities for boring evenings, too many repetitive conversations, too many stores, too many things to buy, too many restaurants . . . it is too easy to say yes when you want to say no.

Limey was able to say no. Limey was selective, he picked and chose out of all the riches only what he knew he wanted and ignored the rest. Of course, this made for clashes between us—"You are too rigid," I yelled—yet now that he is gone, and I do not have him here to counterbalance my childish fear of missing something— "Everyone is at the party but me"—I have finally learned that I was defending something I no longer believed or needed. He was so right. How lucky I am that in spite of my yelling and verbal resistance Limey's influence had actually been working all the while, so that now that I am alone, I think, I hope, I can avoid getting caught up in the sad routine of "filling time" because I am alone. That, to me, is a dangerous hazard of aloneness. When many people talk about independence, they usually seem to have in mind earning money, asserting one's rights, not following the mob, but to me the test of independence is the ability to be alone. Not that one should be a hermit, or antisocial, yet the very idea of aloneness, in our society of two-by-two, arouses pity. "You're all alone in that house?" People look at me as if I'm a bit strange.

To live alone is not, and never was, my choice. I left my father's house for a young marriage, and I never lived alone at any time in my life until now. What is more, I was always the central person in someone else's life—my parents, my husbands, lovers . . . there was always someone to whom I was central and who was central to me. To be without that, no matter how many people there are around, is to be alone. I am peripheral even to those dearest to me, my sons and their families.

It is not an enviable place to be. And yet the very fact that one is able to manage, and even to find some pleasure when alone, to select the friends one wants to see—not to settle for just anyone for company—to choose the things one wants to do—not just for the sake of doing something —implies a growing process that brings with it its own satisfaction and even a sense of pride. And dammit, I want Limey to be proud of me.

That sounds foolish because Limey is dead. And I do not believe there is a life after death. Yet I am not absolutely sure. Not that I believe there is a place where the souls of the dead gather, or that their ghost figures commune, yet there is something that is crying to be kept alive—and I suppose there is the desperate need to believe that no one, even those who were not war heroes, ever lived in vain. Limey was here for seventy-one, almost seventy-two years; what he stood for and what he left behind has value, and I do not want it lost. And since I happen to believe that my behavior reflects his values as much as my own, his standards have become merged with mine. So some part of him still exists in me.

I like that. I like the idea that that man up on the hill, where the boys and I one day scattered his ashes, is still telling me what to do. I like to think that I hear him telling me, "Hila, don't be so impatient, read over what you've written carefully before you send it out . . . Chop the celery fine, not so coarsely . . . Write your angry letter but don't mail it. . . . You have to pick vegetables when they're ready, not tomorrow or the day after . . ." And sometimes I can hear him say, "Hila, I love you." That is the most important of all. I am a woman who was loved and no one can ever take that away from me. I cannot feel deprived.

And yet when I take his advice, and I read this book over carefully, I am stunned by the fact that he can never read it. This is Limey's book, and he cannot give it the finishing touch of his critical eye: he is not here to catch my awkward sentences, my solecisms, my sentences that end in prepositions—he is not here, sitting in his arm-chair, to say, "Don't bother me, I'm reading an interesting book. It reads well, but . . ."

His absence is an amputation and one I cannot get used to. It is hard to get through my head that I will never see Limey again. A widow friend says, "No one understands who hasn't been where we are," and we nod our heads wisely. But what's the good of so much understanding? we ask—we'll go to our graves being understanding women. So what?

Widow. I do not like the word. It is a word that has the sound of pity in it, of hopeless sadness, something like the leftover appendage of someone else. My three-year-old granddaughter looked at me the other day when I was standing naked in front of her, and said, "You are a woman." I laughed at her solemn pronouncement and it pleased me. I am a woman, now, perhaps for the first time, without any label. Neither teen-ager, nor matron, nor wife, nor, God forbid, Senior Citizen (a label I detest)—a mother and a grandmother, yes (those two I don't mind)—but basically I want to exist now as an individual, a woman, not a widow. I want to be a whole person, not the left-behind half of a couple, and I think that wholeness can be achieved because it will be made up, in part, of what Limey gave me.

I had a notion, when I started to write this book, that somewhere along the way I would deal with death. But I have discovered that you do not deal with death—death deals with you. You have to deal with life. And to deal with life one must accept change. I realize that my tendency has been, since Limey died, to hang on to his ways, to make his way my own. A great deal of that is all to the good, and to my advantage, but there is the danger of going overboard in that direction. Hanging on is one thing, but now I must also learn to let go.

Not long ago I said to our son Jimmy, "Someday I

would like to make a little swimming pool in the brook, but Limey would hate it."

Jimmy looked at me sharply. "Dad is dead and you are alive. Do what *you* want."

Of course he was right. The great difficulty is to even know what you want. You are walking gingerly in new territory, in some ways like an adolescent again in search of her identity. So many of the things you did before, so many of the decisions made, were made either in agreement with or in resistance to another person. No decision was made without the impact of Limey's influence. There was always an interaction with someone else, an ever-present emotional reaction and involvement that affected everything you did, and with that gone what you do matters so much less. The loss of that feedback, however, has a certain value: a new process of self-analysis, a new objectivity in discovering what you like or dislike, what you want or reject. I realize now how often I was reacting to Limey rather than making a free, independent choice. If he said black, I might hastily have said white, reacting not to the color, but to so many subjective factors—a tone of voice, a look, a recent quarrel. He could do the same, and did. I think we were no different from any other two people locked into a close, emotional relationship, reacting not to a situation or an object, but to the ambiance of the moment between us.

What I do miss is the intensity of feeling that was the substance of my life, of our life together. Limey was a verification of myself, someone who defined my personality, my every mood. His presence was there to let me know if I was kind or bitchy, witty or foolish, attractive or haggard, gay or depressing. I have no mirror now to let me know. I have no audience, and all I ever needed was an audience of one who, whether he applauded or scowled, never ceased to be totally engaged in my performance.

I must stop saving all the little tidbits of the day to tell Limey. I almost started to cut out a clipping from the *New York Times* for him. It was about Joe's Restaurant on MacDougal Street, "the best Italian restaurant around," Limey used to say. He would have been amused to read that Craig Claiborne finally discovered it and gave it two stars. "It will be ruined now, though," Limey would say.

Friends are fooled by my sturdiness; at least it seems that way to me. While I want no one's pity, the truth is that I am more vulnerable than I was before. Why not? I always had Limey there to comfort me, to calm my anger, to help me pay no attention when someone hurt me, and because I had him those hurts didn't matter so much. But now I feel defenseless, not because I am weak or a woman, but because I am exposed to the world without the emotional protection that he gave me.

I have to find that for myself. And I am learning. I do not look for any big, dramatic change in my life. I never believed that a change in geography, for instance, was very useful. But I am learning that it is important, helpful, to experiment, to be open to new experiences, not to be rigid in sticking to a familiar pattern. There will be hits and misses. To live is to be open to life, not to be afraid to take a chance. I am on the threshold of a new phase in my life, and perhaps it is just as well that I have neither crystal ball nor blueprint. Maybe it will be fun to see what happens.

I have had difficulty in getting past the year of Limey's illness. I keep thinking of him lying in bed, or sitting in the wheelchair, when I want to remember the good times. My widow friends tell me that that will come, and now I consciously try to reconstruct them. I want to remember the supper picnics on the beach at the Cape with all the kids and all the grown-ups, and the sleigh-riding parties at Diane's house, the campfires at the falls, and consuming endless martinis at Pete's Bar, and always the joy of coming home after a trip—"It's so good to be home, we had a lovely time but it's so nice to be here." I want to remember Limey staying up all one Christmas Eve putting together a wagon for Jonny, Limey loving his new shirt from L. L. Bean's, Limey bringing me the first ripe tomato from the garden—Limey, Limey.

I hope the memory of the last terrible year will fade and the rest remain, and yet somehow I don't want that to happen either. It was too deeply searing an emotional experience, the deepest of my life, and that must have some value. I have been asked what did I do that was right or wrong, what advice can I give to someone else. I can't. There were no intellectual decisions, it was all gut feeling, and I guess that is all the advice I can offer. I had to do what I *felt* was right, I had to trust my love for Limey and my own need for survival, and those are emotional choices that I do not believe are unsound. I married Limey because I fell in love, not because he was "a good catch" or for convenience or for any thought-out, deliberated reasons. I was wildly in love. Those instincts then were right. I could not have made a better choice for myself, even though we did not have what anyone could describe as "a perfect marriage." I don't know what a perfect marriage is. Ours had despair and joy and anger and love, and rough times and tenderness—and our last year together had all of those same emotions intensified a hundred times. There was no right and wrong. It was a year in which the smallest fluctuation on the emotional scale was enormously magnified and was a further learning, molding, developing force for experiencing life. Why should I want to forget that? I don't.

I do know one thing: whatever I did for Limey that last year of his life to make it a little more bearable for him had nothing to do with the fact that I am a woman and he a man. Some people have said to me, "A woman can manage these things better." I cannot agree. I *know* Limey would have done the same for me. Limey was capable of great love and he would have been sensitive to my needs, as I tried to be to his, and somehow managed. I cannot imagine any other way.

Every different part of my life in the past had its own joys as well as its problems, so it is not unrealistic to believe that the future will bring its own pleasures. I would be stupid to rule out the possibility. Of course I get depressed, and I want to close myself in, but what a be-

trayal that would be. "Don't mourn for me," Limey said.
"Have a good time."

I think Pushkin wrote the lines:

> Never say with grief he is no more,
> But rather say with thankfulness he was.

Hila Colman

HILA COLMAN is the author of fifty published books including *The Girl from Puerto Rico* (*1961*); *Classmates by Request* (*1964*); *Mixed Marriage Daughter* (*1968*); *Claudia, Where Are You* (*1969*); *Diary of a Frantic Kid Sister* (*1973*); *After the Wedding* (*1975*); *Nobody Has to Be a Kid Forever* (*1976*); and *The Amazing Miss Laura* (*1976*). About the last, *Publishers Weekly* has said: "Without heavy moralizing, Colman delivers a meaningful story. . . . Her new story, like the earlier works, has a sound grounding in social prospects and problems."